A Look Inside Alzheimer's

A Look Inside Alzheimer's

Marjorie N. Allen

Susan Dublin, RN

Patricia J. Kimmerly

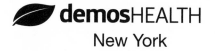
New York

Visit our website at www.demoshealth.com

ISBN: 978-1-936303-46-5
e-book ISBN: 978-1-617051-47-0

Acquisitions Editor: Noreen Henson
Compositor: diacriTech

Medical information provided by Demos Health, in the absence of a visit with a health care professional, must be considered as an educational service only. This book is not designed to replace a physician's independent judgment about the appropriateness or risks of a procedure or therapy for a given patient. Our purpose is to provide you with information that will help you make your own health care decisions.

The information and opinions provided here are believed to be accurate and sound, based on the best judgment available to the authors, editors, and publisher, but readers who fail to consult appropriate health authorities assume the risk of injuries. The publisher is not responsible for errors or omissions. The editors and publisher welcome any reader to report to the publisher any discrepancies or inaccuracies noticed.

Library of Congress Cataloging-in-Publication Data
Allen, Marjorie N. (Majorie Nicholson), 1931–
  A look inside Alzheimer's disease / by Marjorie N. Allen, Susan Dublin, Patricia J. Kimmerly.
    p. cm.
  Includes bibliographical references and index.
  ISBN 978-1-936303-46-5 (alk. paper)
  1. Alzheimer's disease. I. Dublin, Susan. II. Kimmerly, Patricia J. III. Title.
  RC523.A3627 2013
  616.8'31—dc23
                    2012021198

Special discounts on bulk quantities of Demos Health books are available to corporations, professional associations, pharmaceutical companies, health care organizations, and other qualifying groups. For details, please contact:

Special Sales Department
Demos Medical Publishing, LLC
11 West 42nd Street, 15th Floor
New York, NY 10036
Phone: 800-532-8663 or 212-683-0072
Fax: 212-941-7842
E-mail: rsantana@demosmedpub.com

Printed in the United States of America by Hamilton Printing
12 13 14 15 / 5 4 3 2 1

In Loving Memory
Dave, Mary, Daws, and Char

Contents

Foreword

Mixing one part guide for living with Alzheimer's disease, one part scientific background and one part first-hand vignettes from their own experiences, Marjorie Allen, Susan Dublin and PJ Kimmerly have created something truly useful to those dealing with Alzheimer's, their caregivers, and their treaters. This guide contains both a wonderful resource of information as well as a moving, first-person account of dealing with memory loss and other symptoms of Alzheimer's disease. The writers demonstrate how this disease may affect the memory but doesn't touch the core humanity in all of us. With wonderful references and resources, this work shows what is it like to live with this disease and, even more importantly, live well in spite of this disease. Practical and important questions about finances, care, and relationships are dealt with directly. At the same time, humor and compassion flow throughout this work as we all (patients, families, and health care professionals) do the best we can when faced with challenges we sometimes think we can't overcome. But overcome them we do, one step at a time. And those steps are made all the easier with guides like these.

Daniel Z. Press, MD
Assistant Professor of Neurology
Harvard Medical School

Preface

When I lost my husband, Dave, to Alzheimer's disease (AD) three years ago, I never expected to hear from his niece, Sue Dublin, that she had been diagnosed with AD at the age of 52. This was a wakeup call about a disease I really knew little about, even though my husband had it. He died six months after he was diagnosed. I ran across a novel called *Still Alice* by Lisa Genova that told the story of a woman with early onset Alzheimer's from the first sign until the end. Although Genova did not have AD, she created an exceptionally believable character that did. I read it, was enthralled by it, and mailed it to Sue.

She loved it and said she wanted more than anything to write a book with me and her friend PJ Kimmerly, who also had early stage, to help the public better understand how much those in the early stages of the disease want to be treated as viable personalities who are able to interact with others. I agreed, and *A Look Inside Alzheimer's* is the result. The book is a clear indication that these two women have a lot to say about their disease. Shortly before we began this book, Sue was interviewed by Jasmyn Belcher at WRVO public radio in March 2010 regarding her diagnosis of Alzheimer's at such a young age. The interview was picked up nationally, and that's how friends of hers in Washington State found out she had Alzheimer's and gave her a call.

When the signs we associate with Alzheimer's disease are present, why can't the doctor suggest the possibility with ways to deal with cognitive problems and then go ahead with tests, understanding that AD might be the final diagnosis anyway? This is a disease that must be understood. It is life changing and requires a new way of living a day at a time. It is ultimately connected to the aging process and there are certain inevitable developments that lead to the inability of a person to care for himself or herself, but meeting the disease head-on before this happens is one way to find out more about the disease from a person who has it.

There seems to be a debate about whether there is a lasting emotional connection between those with Alzheimer's and those who care for them. Sue and PJ definitely feel that connection to family and friends and I invite you to get to know them in this book. Also, I never doubted the love between my husband and me, even at the end.

Marjorie N. Allen

Acknowledgments

While writing this book, we received a great deal of valuable help from family members, as well as from the Central New York Alzheimer's Association website, which was updated often and offered current advances in Alzheimer's. Thanks also to our editor Noreen Henson, who guided us through the writing of this book and helped us through the rough spots. We further wish to thank Sue's neurologist Dr. Daniel Press for his care and understanding and for agreeing to write the Foreword for the book. Also, thanks to the staff at Hillcrest Commons in Pittsfield, MA, for making my husband Dave Allen's temporary stay there as comfortable as possible. Sue and PJ met each other at the Central New York Alzheimer's Association Chapter in Syracuse, New York. I am also grateful for all the help I received from Bea Cowlin, facilitator of the local Alzheimer's caregiver group after Dave was diagnosed.

Grateful acknowledgment is also extended to the following for permission to reproduce some of the content in the book: Ashley LeBeau, Assistant Administrator of Hillcrest Commons, for providing the photo of the Hillcrest Commons staff; Robert G. Nassau, Associate Director, Office of Clinical Legal Education at Syracuse University, for permission to reprint the photo of Sue and PJ; and *The Berkshire Eagle* of Pittsfield, Massachusetts, for permission to reprint the article that serves as the Appendix.

Marjorie N. Allen

Susan Dublin

PJ Kimmerly

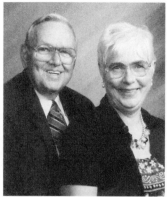

Dave & Marge (Early Stage)

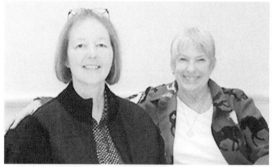

Sue and PJ

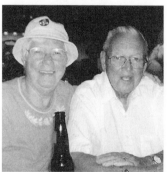

Marge & Dave (Later Stage)

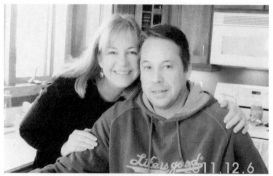

PJ's Children Tiffany and Char

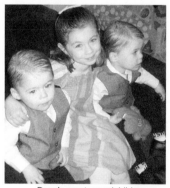

Dave's great-grandchildren
Demetri & Dante (twins) and Aniya

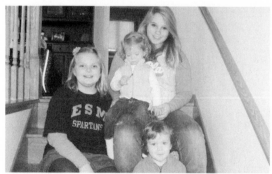

PJ's grandchildren
Jenna, Lauren, Jack, and Ella

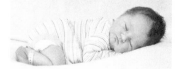

Abigail – Sue's granddaughter

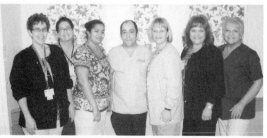

Hillcrest Commons Staff

Introduction

*A*lzheimer's is only one form of dementia. There are several kinds of cognitive dementia and each has its own set of symptoms. The main problem, however, is that once a person is diagnosed, there is no cure as yet, and it will just get progressively worse.

Alzheimer's is an incurable disease that can begin at any age. In the meantime, those with the disease who show symptoms before they are eligible for Medicare or aren't yet eligible for Social Security are faced with financial difficulties and have to go through a change of lifestyle in which they lose their independence along with their jobs. Those in the late stages of the disease are apt to need care 24-7 with a major increase in medical costs. The outcome so far is bleak, even with an increase in research. Those with early onset will ultimately reach the final stages of the disease. At present, it's a matter of accepting the inevitable and finding the routine that will allow appreciation of what life offers.

This book basically covers Alzheimer's disease (AD) and the way in which society here and abroad is impacted, with feedback from two women—Sue Dublin and PJ Kimmerly—who have been diagnosed before the disease has overwhelmed them, and from my own efforts in dealing with my husband's increasing symptoms over the last year of his life. We started writing this book in September 2010. Since then, more and more attention is being paid to find a cure or a way to cope with AD, not just in the United States but internationally as well. Almost everyone knows someone with Alzheimer's disease, but very few understand the disease itself.

Chapter 1 defines the disease called "Alzheimer's" and how the medical community has made an effort to understand it. Chapter 2 incorporates the experiences of Sue, PJ, and my husband, Dave, as we all were faced with unusual symptoms and no answers as to what was causing them. Chapter 3 speaks about the way in which the diagnosis affects the interactions between family and friends and coming to terms with life changes that must be faced. Chapter 4 outlines the need to plan for a new lifestyle when the diagnosis makes the future uncertain. Chapter 5 offers ways in which we all tried to develop a routine that incorporated AD into our daily lives. Chapter 6 is a collection of the ways in which family and friends can try to accept the reality of AD and how it has impacted them. Chapter 7 offers stories from later in the disease process. Chapter 8 talks about the options offered to patients and their caregivers as to how best to deal with the disease with different resources such as support groups, organizations, and trials and studies. Chapter 9 covers the latest findings on AD as well as how to face the future here and abroad. The Appendix is a reprint of an article that appeared in *The Berkshire Eagle* over 20 years ago called "Growing Old: Independence Fading."

Resources are listed as support groups, organizations, and trials and studies. The glossary defines many of the terms used in the field of AD and other dementias, and there is a Further Reading list to supplement the bibliographic listings in many of the chapters.

What Is Alzheimer's Disease?

Alzheimer's is a phantom disease. There are no specific tests that offer an immediate diagnosis for this type of dementia. And there is still no cure. Once the diagnosis is made, the waiting game begins. The symptoms are progressive and varied and accelerate, sometimes quickly, as in Creutzfeldt-Jakob disease or vascular dementia, and sometimes over a period of many years, as in general Alzheimer's disease (AD). Unfortunately, according to research by neurologist Jon Glass, the frequency of "treatable" causes of dementia is only 20% of all dementias, and AD is not a treatable cause. It is estimated that 5.4 million Americans live with AD, that every 70 seconds someone is being diagnosed, and we know the incidence of early onset Alzheimer's (before age 65) is increasing.

A SHORT HISTORY OF ALZHEIMER'S DISEASE

In 1906, Dr. Alois Alzheimer, a German physician, noticed dense deposits surrounding the nerve cells in the brain while performing an autopsy on a patient who had suffered from

severe memory problems, confusion, and difficulty understanding questions for many years. This abnormality, only
identifiable after death, would later be named Alzheimer's
disease by psychiatrist Emil Kraepelin.

In the 1960s, the medical community formally recognized AD as a disease, and not a normal part of aging. This
is when they first discovered a link between cognitive decline
and the number of plaques and tangles in the brain. In the
1970s, AD became a significant area of research. In a 1976 editorial, neurologist Dr. Robert Katzman, founding member of
the Alzheimer's Association, characterized Alzheimer's as a
major killer and a significant public health problem. It had
previously been considered a rare condition, but Katzman's
editorial brought the disease out of obscurity and into the
forefront of medical scientific research. In the 1990s, several
drugs were approved to treat the cognitive symptoms of the
disease, with Aricept and Namenda the most commonly prescribed. According to the Research Center of the Alzheimer's
Association, "although there is no cure, Alzheimer's medications can temporarily slow the worsening of symptoms and
improve quality of life for those with Alzheimer's and their
caregivers."

In the 21st century, more and more attention is being paid
to AD with a debate at present about whether a person with
Alzheimer's loses identity and can be considered "gone" at some
point in the disease. This book will attempt to show the inner
thoughts of those who have AD and the connection that remains
no matter how long the disease continues. It is a matter of deep
concern that so many doctors in our society are unaware of or
dismiss the signs of AD and spend far too much time looking
for alternate diagnoses. For the patient, this long-term search is
exhausting and frustrating, and by the time AD becomes the only
reasonable diagnosis, the patient is actually relieved to hear the
news, as devastating as it is. For age-related AD, doctors focus on
medical problems and avoid even discussing the possibility that
a patient might be in the beginning stages of AD, or could contribute personally to understanding if only the diagnosis were
recognized earlier and the right questions were asked.

MISCONCEPTIONS ABOUT ALZHEIMER'S DISEASE

Again, before the 21st century, AD was not an accepted diagnosis. It was well known that older people in their 70s, 80s, and 90s were apt to show signs of dementia, but no one talked about it because it was considered a mental illness. Early onset was completely unknown. If people were demented, they were considered insane, but AD is a form of dementia and dementia is not insanity. It is a neurological disease. There are medications that help certain symptoms but cannot cure AD, and there are trial studies looking at other ways to treat and eventually cure the disease. Those who have AD often have to wait months or even years for a diagnosis, while every other conceivable illness is ruled out—"It can't be Alzheimer's. You're too young," or "You don't have Alzheimer's. Your problems are health related." Granted, there is no way at present to be sure of the diagnosis, but if the possibility is raised based on symptoms at the outset, other illnesses can still be ruled out. In the meantime, people could better understand what might be happening to them. The truth is, many general practitioners are reluctant to share a diagnosis such as Alzheimer's.

The following suggestions offer ways in which the medical community can help their patients understand what they might be facing, at least in the early stages, of AD:

- Many family physicians are apt to dismiss symptoms of dementia in its beginning stages. The earlier the disease is recognized, the sooner treatment can be started.
- It is important for social workers and private health aides to realize that the patient understands a great deal but cannot always communicate clearly. Patience is necessary.
- Patients often become frustrated and angry when a caregiver insists they pursue certain activities. It is important not to argue with a patient who is being unreasonable.
- When a patient wants you to do something that cannot be done, agree but postpone any action. They probably won't remember what seemed so important at the time.

- Finally, a person with AD needs a routine, even though it will periodically have to be changed as the disease progresses.

The physical body breaks down as a person ages, and with new ways to treat many diseases, people are living longer. That, plus the large number of "baby boomers," including those born before 1961, increases the number of people who might face cognitive problems---people like Sue and PJ, as well as my husband, Dave.

DEMENTIA IN ALL ITS FORMS

The public sees AD as a singular disease, but the truth is that there are several different kinds of AD, with a common base of dementia. Alzheimer's comprises 50% to 80% of dementia cases. Below, according to Jon Glass, are types of dementia that might or might not lead to AD:

Cortical dementia is a disorder affecting the cerebral cortex, the outer area of the brain dealing with thinking abilities like memory and language. AD and Creutzfeldt-Jakob disease (a rapidly fatal disorder) are two forms of cortical dementia in which people typically show severe memory loss and aphasia—the inability to recall words and understand language. Another rare form of Alzheimer's is Posterior Cortical Atrophy, which affects vision.

Subcortical dementia is a dysfunction in parts of the brain beneath the cortex. Usually, forgetfulness and language difficulties are not present. People with subcortical dementia such as Parkinson's dementia, Huntington's disease, AIDS dementia complex, and some types of multiple sclerosis (MS) tend to show changes in speed of thinking and ability to initiate activities.

Multi-infarct dementia (MID) is a vascular disorder that affects both parts of the brain and is caused by a small series of strokes. Symptoms of dementia in any one person may be caused by either AD or MID or both. The symptoms for each problem are very similar, and MID may be a risk factor for AD.

Dementia with Lewy Bodies is a disorder in which alertness and severity of cognitive symptoms may fluctuate daily. Visual hallucinations, muscle rigidity, and tremors are common.

Frontotemporal dementia is a disorder in which nerve cells in the front and side regions of the brain are especially affected. Typical symptoms include changes in personality and behavior and difficulty with language. Pick's disease is a frontotemporal dementia that tends to affect only certain areas of the brain.

According to an overview of AD by the Alzheimer's Association, although a diagnosis of AD was first identified more than 100 years ago, research into the disease has only gained momentum in the last 30 years. With the exception of certain inherited forms of the disease, the cause or causes remain unknown. Studies show that brain changes in individuals with Alzheimer's are thought to begin 10 years or more before such symptoms as memory loss appear. A new diagnostic category representing the earliest changes is called "preclinical Alzheimer's disease." Biomarkers being considered are brain volume, level of glucose metabolism and levels of beta-amyloid in the brain, and levels of beta-amyloid and tau in cerebrospinal fluid. Scientists in Spain, according to the Press Association, have developed a blood test that identifies AD in its earliest stages and would give non-specialists a tool for this very hard-to-diagnose disease. The test can predict early stage Alzheimer's when there is a buildup of amyloid beta in the brains of patients with cognitive impairment. It means that people like Sue and PJ wouldn't have to wait for months or years to find out whether they do or do not have the disease. The United States and the United Kingdom are also involved in research regarding a potential blood test that diagnoses the possibility of dementia. Medical correspondent Stephen Adams of the *Telegraph* quotes Dr. Anne Corbett of the Alzheimer's Society as saying, "One in three people over 65 will die with dementia, yet dementia research is still drastically under-funded." Also, there are trials being conducted on medications that appear to attack the brain and actually replace the damage that AD causes. Work is being done to fight the disease, but it takes time, and many people now being diagnosed may not be able to take advantage of success in the field. With a rapidly aging baby boomer population, AD will continue to impact more lives. From 2000 to 2006, deaths from AD increased 46.1%, while other selected causes of death decreased. Strategic investments in other diseases have resulted in declines in deaths, and the same type of investment for AD is needed.

For those who have not yet been diagnosed with AD, there are certain signs and symptoms that should have been obvious to the general practitioner, even though the doctor might not have a great deal of knowledge about the disease. Unlike many incurable diseases, Alzheimer's is more cognitive than physical in its early stages, and so far there is no way to control it or prevent it and no way to actually diagnose it until after death. As of now, there is no way to stop the disease. It is progressive.

Until a fully acceptable test is available that can determine specifically that a patient has Alzheimer's or may be at risk for the disease, those with AD may have to spend a year or more waiting for a diagnosis before every other disease is ruled out.

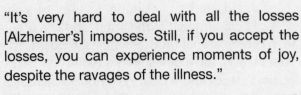

"It's very hard to deal with all the losses [Alzheimer's] imposes. Still, if you accept the losses, you can experience moments of joy, despite the ravages of the illness."

(CASTLEMAN ET AL., p. 294)

According to Stephen McConnell, vice president for policy at the Alzheimer's Association, "people with midlife Alzheimer's often are fired or are forced to take early retirement. They can lose their health insurance, and they either don't qualify for or have trouble applying for government programs designed to help the elderly." In the last ten years, AD has become the subject of numerous books, almost all of them from the viewpoint of a caregiver. Unfortunately, there is an assumption that if a person has AD, even early onset, that person would not be able to write a book about the development of the disease. This is not at all true. Although AD affects each individual differently, there are enough common symptoms to indicate at least a probable diagnosis of AD. The two women who are sharing their experiences in this book have been diagnosed with midlife AD and want to educate the public on the workings of this disease. My husband, Dave, had the more common form of Alzheimer's coupled with myriad physical problems, but this book will include my experiences and offer guidelines on understanding all types of Alzheimer's. The development of the disease is inevitable and, as time goes on, the toll it takes is evident. The sooner a diagnosis is made, the sooner coping mechanisms can be instituted.

SYMPTOMS RELATED TO AD

Presently, the diagnosis of AD is based on certain symptoms that are considered indicative of the disease. When these symptoms appear in someone under 70, it doesn't seem likely that the diagnosis of Alzheimer's is the correct diagnosis and much time is spent ruling out everything except Alzheimer's. If there is anything positive about having early stage AD, it is that the symptoms at first are mild and intermittent. In other words, some days are better than others. A person with the disease in this stage is able to share a great deal of information about what is happening. Below, according to Darby Morhardt of *USA Today*, is a list of symptoms that are simply age-related and those that might indicate Alzheimer's.

What's Normal	What's Not
Sometimes forgetting why you came into a room or what you planned to say	Problems staying organized day to day, losing track of steps in making a call or playing a game
Sometimes grasping for the right word	Forgetting simple words more often
Misplacing keys and wallets	Putting things in unusual places, like a watch in the sugar bowl
Trouble balancing a checkbook at times	Paying bills twice or not at all

These are only a few of the symptoms that might indicate AD, but any of the above abnormal symptoms call for further investigation. This is a book for families, as well as members of the medical community. The idea that those with the disease lose their sense of self is wrong. The emotional connection between those living with the disease and their loved ones is never lost and becomes more evident as time goes on.

Alzheimer's is a disease that could and might very well be passed down to younger members of a family when they are older. This book utilizes diary entries and correspondence tapes from those with AD as well as from relatives and caregivers, and included in these stories are humor, pathos, and honesty, offering understanding and ability to cope as the disease progresses.

As of March 2010, the Alzheimer's Association reported that 5.2 million Americans had been diagnosed with AD in all its forms. A more recent study in 2011, however, expands the number to 5.4 million. Now is the time to focus on understanding the disease better and learning to deal on a day to day level with it, and if not to find a cure, at least to find a way to slow its progression, while accepting the inevitable change in lifestyle until a cure is found. According to the 2011 report, by 2029, all baby boomers will be at least 65 years old. Those in the early stages still have the ability to share a great deal. As time goes on, more and more people with the disease can offer the insight needed to help families cope with the disease and by doing so will no longer feel so alone.

IMPACT OF ALZHEIMER'S DISEASE ON SOCIETY

Every 70 seconds, someone in America develops AD, and by 2050 that time is expected to be every 33 seconds. Over the coming decades, the baby boom population is projected to add 10 million people to these numbers. In 2050, the incidence of AD is expected to approach nearly a million people per year, with a total estimated prevalence of 11 to 16 million people. Dramatic increases in the population of people living longer across all racial and ethnic groups will also significantly affect the numbers of people living with AD.

SEPARATING THE HUMAN BEING FROM THE DISEASE

Importantly, there has also been a debate about whether a person with Alzheimer's loses identity and can be considered "gone" at some point in the disease. It is a matter of deep concern that so many doctors in our society are unaware of or dismiss the signs of AD and spend far too much time looking for alternate diagnoses. For the person living with AD, this long-term search is exhausting and frustrating, and by the time Alzheimer's becomes the only reasonable diagnosis, some people are actually relieved to hear the news, as devastating as it is. Doctors tend to focus on medical problems and avoid even discussing the possibility that a person might be in the beginning stages of AD. Many people would be helped if the right questions were asked and they were diagnosed earlier.

It is important to educate people that AD is not a loss of self. It is a gradual change in self that eventually affects the physical and cognitive abilities but retains the inner emotional connection. Even though in the later stages of the disease the loved one may not be able to give a name to the caregiver, the connection is still there. When someone like evangelist Pat Robertson encourages a partner to divorce if his spouse has Alzheimer's because she is "gone," or a journalist such as Barry Peterson writes a book to convince the public he is justified in having a new partner because his wife who is in a nursing home is "gone," the public is not well served. Also, the decisions made by these people are about a man whose wife has dementia, not a woman whose husband has dementia, but either way, this has become a serious bone of contention for many people dealing with AD in their families. Author Elizabeth Tierney in *Dignifying Dementia* makes it very clear that she never gave up on her husband, staying with him until the end.

It is important to educate people that AD is not a loss of self. It is a gradual change in self that eventually affects the physical and cognitive abilities but retains the inner emotional connection.

It is never easy to deal with the changes that occur, but accepting the losses and setting up a new routine whenever necessary, as well as allowing others, family or friends, to help out when feasible, will make a caregiver's life more stress-free. In addition, with a predictable routine, the patient will be more capable of accepting the disease as it progresses.

BIBLIOGRAPHY

Adams, Stephen. 2012. "Blood Test to Detect Early Stages of Alzheimer's."*The Telegraph.*

Alzheimer's Association. 2008. "Founding Association Member Katzman Dies." *Alzheimer's News*, Accessed September 29. http://www.alz.org/news_and_events_Alzheimer_News_9-29-2008.asp.

Alzheimer's Association. 2010. "Alzheimer's Disease Facts and Figures." *Alzheimer's & Dementia: The Journal of the Alzheimer's Association* 6 (2): 158–194.

Alzheimer's Association. 2011. "Alzheimer's Disease Facts and Figures." *Alzheimer's & Dementia: The Journal of the Alzheimer's Association* 7 (2): 1–58.

Breen, Tom. 2011. "Pat Robertson Says Alzheimer's Makes Divorce OK." *Associated Press*, Accessed September 15. http://news.yahoo.com/pat-robertson-says-alzheimers-makes-divorce-ok-000952197.html.

Castleman, M., D. Gallagher-Thompson, and M. Naythons. 2000. *There's Still a Person In There: The Complete Guide to Treating and Coping With Alzheimer's*. New York: G.P. Putnam's Sons.

Fackelmann, Kathleen. 2007. "Who Thinks of Alzheimer's in Someone So Young?" *USA Today*, Accessed June 12. http://www.usatoday.com/news/health/2007-06-11-alzheimers-cover_N.htm.

Glass, Jon. 2010. "WebMD: Types of Dementia. Pp 1–2." Accessed March 2. http://www.webmd.com/brain/types-dementia?page=1.

History of Alzheimer's. 2011. "Alzheimer's Disease Research." Accessed September 23. http://www.ahaf.org/alzheimers/about/understanding/history.html.

Morhardt, Darby. 2009. "Alzheimer's: What You Need to Know." *USA Today*, Accessed April 21. http://www.usatoday.com/news/alzheimers.htm.

Research Center of Alzheimer's Association. "Current Alzheimer's Treatments." http://www.alz.org/research/science/alzheimers_disease_treatments.asp#how.

Tierney, Elizabeth. 2011. *Dignifying Dementia*. Ireland: Oak Tree Press.

2
Early Signs

Susan Dublin and her husband, Gary, live in DeWitt, NY, a suburb of Syracuse, and have three children, two married, one in high school—Ben, Kaitie, and Elizabeth (Lizzie). Susan is in her early fifties and the diagnosis of Alzheimer's has drastically changed the family's plans for the future. The following pages are Sue's experiences in looking for a diagnosis.

EARLY SIGNS—SUE

Welcome to my world. My name is Sue Dublin, and when I was 52 years old I was diagnosed with Alzheimer's disease (AD). For the past few years, I have been struggling with how to deal with this diagnosis. However, the time leading up to a diagnosis was perhaps even more difficult and frustrating because doctors avoided the possibility that someone as young as I was, just entering my 50s, actually had Alzheimer's. Therefore, upsetting things were happening to me and I didn't have the slightest idea why.

Basically, in every speech, article, or event in which I now discuss the onset of the disease, one question always comes up,

"What was the first sign of the disease for you?" The answer, for me, was having trouble using an escalator. I couldn't bring myself to step on a stair that was constantly moving. That was the first spatial issue I could not overcome. I didn't realize what that meant at the time. I had to find places that had elevators or stairs. Some elevators were freight elevators and in some places they were used so infrequently they were filthy dirty. Using stairs was great, except when my appointment was on the 10th floor.

Another early sign was when my husband, Gary, and I were on a trip and staying in a hotel. You could either walk upstairs or you could go on the elevator, and everyone went in different ways because they were going up to their rooms. I got disoriented, not realizing what was going on. All I knew was I couldn't catch up and I couldn't figure out from where I was sitting on a balcony how to get back to the room. It took what seemed like a very long time for Gary to realize I wasn't around and all of a sudden there he was. Quite frankly, at the time I thought it was quite funny. I just sat right there on the balcony and knew eventually someone would come. When Gary did come, it turned out I was really right on top of the room. I couldn't figure that out. And again, you know, it's something you wouldn't think about, but it was probably the early part of Alzheimer's, way back before such symptoms were obvious, and that's one of the problems. There are no specific guidelines. There are some, but everybody seems to have different problems.

Yet another earlier sign was that when we went on vacation, Gary and I always did crossword puzzles. We'd both do the answers and I'd write in the box. But this time, I tried to put the answer in the box in the right spot in the crossword puzzle, and I couldn't get it in the right way. Gary got very frustrated and actually kind of angry that I wasn't putting it in the right way. I just couldn't do it. Neither of us had any idea then why, but that is what happened. These situations were stressful for both of us.

The Meaning of Friendship

Two of my special friends, Lee Ann and Anne, were always there for me during this time. It was helpful to know I could call them. Half the time I would pick up the phone and call just to have support and other times just to tell and to share what was going on. Knowing there is a problem and not knowing why is devastating. When I finally was diagnosed, although it was not a diagnosis anyone would want, it was actually a relief to finally know why these things were happening. Also, through my research into the disease online, I joined a support group and met PJ, my counterpart in this book.

My Story

Long before I had any idea what the future might bring, I was actively involved in health care. I started my career after receiving my bachelor's degree in nursing from Hartwick College in Oneonta, New York, in 1977. My first job was at Crouse Irving Hospital in Syracuse. I worked on a medical floor where I was a staff nurse, also in a rotation as charge nurse. After a year in the hospital, I decided I wanted different experiences, so I applied for a Public Health nurse position in Madison County. There, I was responsible for calling on elderly people to monitor their condition and evaluate their status. I also made "well visits" to new mothers after they were released from the hospital. I educated them on the care of a new baby.

I developed a program for better continuity for teenage pregnancies within the county. I would establish the teens with local OBGYNs and go with them on appointments, then follow up weekly, making sure they were staying on task. I developed lasting relationships with the new moms. I developed and ran expectant parents' classes evenings to help with early parenting issues and care. I trained and certified Home Health Aides.

I left my Public Health position to raise a family after three years. Gary and I were married right out of college in 1977. After Ben was born and before Kaitie showed up, we moved back to Syracuse. I worked nights doing private duty nursing for the elderly while Gary watched Ben and ultimately Kaitie. During that time I also worked part-time at Hill Haven Nursing Home nights and weekends as "charge nurse." I really loved working with the elderly; their humor was wonderful and they were so grateful for anything you did for them. The wonderful relationships and the age of my patients led to an overwhelming amount of homemade Afghans that are still around my house.

When Kaitie was 6, I went to Lyndon Pediatrics as a nurse. Lyndon was our pediatrician's office and I liked the way it was run. During my 19 years at Lyndon, I was a nurse and, for a period of time, nurse manager. In addition to my nursing duties, I was responsible for scheduling, triage, interviewing, hiring and training new nurses, and educating parents.

Facing the Inevitable

A few years ago, I started having problems at work. This was before my diagnosis. I'd worked in that office for so many years, it was obvious that I was experienced and had no problems doing my job. I was in charge of making out schedules for the staff and that type of thing, but one time I wrote the year way, way out and one of the nurses said, "I don't think I'd be around then." I know she was kidding, but I looked at the calendar and to me it looked fine. I couldn't figure out what she was even talking about. Then I got that hot, warm feeling like I'm doing something stupid, but I didn't know what it was, and that was very upsetting. I went out and got a new calendar watch to see if that made it better. For a while, to some degree, it actually did.

According to Stephen McConnell, vice president for policy at Alzheimer's Association, "People with midlife Alzheimer's often are fired or are forced to take early retirement. They can lose their health insurance and they either don't qualify for or have trouble applying for government programs designed to help the elderly."

(FACKELMANN, 2007)

Back at the office, we had to enter information, but I wouldn't write it in exactly the right spot—again, probably spatial issues, entering things that didn't belong where they were entered. I started noticing that there were changes in how I was doing my job. I had other people cover for me so that I wasn't doing direct patient care. It was hard to pass on numerous responsibilities. I was aware of people watching to see what I was doing because no one understood just what was going on. The more someone watched me the more uncomfortable I got, coming up from that hot place, making me even more uncomfortable, and obviously, something was wrong. Our office doctors helped me get an appointment with a neurologist. They were all concerned, and that was very helpful. But at that point, I stopped working. I left my job.

Sharing My Concerns

I told my parents at some point that I was having some problems at work, and that the doctors and I had decided it was time to leave. At home, I couldn't write checks, do simple math, or, being out with a friend, I couldn't figure out the bill and things like that. When I told my mom and dad, they were concerned and glad I was seeing the doctor and anxious every time I went to the doctor to know what was going on. Gary was supportive from the beginning, even though neither of us had any idea what the problem was. Ben and Kaitie were older and on their own, and Lizzie, our youngest, was busy with school activities.

When I did get an appointment with the neurologist, he evaluated and went through all the questions and everything that was going on, did tons of lab work, and ordered a computed tomography scan and magnetic resonance imaging (MRI). I was anxious and queasy about going into the machine, but after he gave me medication to deal with the anxiety, I was fine. The first day, he had me go backwards with numbers, phone numbers, questions to check my orientation, information about Chelsea Clinton, questions like that, where I had a little bit of an issue. He showed me a black and white picture and asked me to find certain things, and he seemed very concerned that I couldn't do so. Later on, during another appointment I went through a lot of testing for memory and thought that I had done extremely poorly and was very worried. I was exhausted from the questions. It was like a computer game and my eyes were tired, and at that point I was thinking, "I don't really care."

17

Misconceptions and No Diagnosis

After a while, I was going every two or four weeks, and still the doctor couldn't come up with what was really going on. There was nothing concrete; they were not typical symptoms for Alzheimer's that he was aware of and nothing was coming together. He thought at one time it might be MS and kept coming back to that. He did a brain scan and spinal tap, thinking that might show something for MS, but it didn't. One thing he did do at the very beginning—it was around Labor Day, I remember—was put me on Aricept right away. He said he didn't know what was going on, but he was going to treat it aggressively. I didn't have trouble tolerating it so he kept me on that medication.

Perhaps one of the most difficult things facing those with early onset is that people don't believe the diagnosis is correct.

Hey, Look at Me—I'm Still Here

One of the things that really bothered me in the beginning with these appointments was that the doctor acted as if I wasn't even there, and that was very frustrating. He was talking to Gary all the time. I didn't really like that very much and talked about it with Gary, and he kind of redirected the doctor so that he was talking to me also. One of the most objectionable reactions other people have when they know you have Alzheimer's is to treat you as if you're in a coma and unable to communicate. Not so. We ran into a similar situation just the other day. I needed new shoes and we went to the SAS shoe store. Gary was helping me try to find something I liked and a shoe salesman came to help too. I was having a bit of trouble finding my words and it wasn't long before the salesman was talking strictly to Gary and not me. The salesman was very nice, but he picked up on something being wrong and pretty much ignored me after that.

Other testing with this doctor included electroencephalography, hearing, and myriad other tests. Nothing showed up that was significant in any of the testing, except the first or second MRI did show some of the plaques on the brain. He said at that time that it might come and go, but we really never discussed it. More tests and more tests. It seemed like they were constant, and he still didn't seem able to diagnose the problem. After one of the tests, he called us when he got the results back, and said, "Great news. Celebrate. All's clear." It wasn't, but at that time, I guess, it was, and that was hopeful. We also tried adding medication, Namenda, but at that time it just didn't work with me, so that was frustrating. I finally asked the doctor if it was appropriate to get a second opinion. He said, "If you were my daughter, I would get a second opinion." I talked to my brother, Doug, and he was able to touch base with a doctor in Boston who specialized in cognitive problems and Alzheimer's, so that's where we went.

The Final Diagnosis

We made an appointment with Dr. Daniel Z. Press, a neurologist at Beth Israel Deaconess Medical Center, Boston, and assistant professor of neurology at Harvard Medical School. My first visit included a complete neurological evaluation. The initial visit was several hours long. We had provided all of the notes and test results from the doctor in Syracuse and Dr. Press reviewed the notes while he was testing me. It was Gary's observation that Dan started with no direction and slowly processed the problem by directing me to my weaknesses. At the end, the doctor knew without a doubt that it was posterior cortical atrophy (PCA). He said it is a very rare form of Alzheimer's, and he only had a few patients with that disease. Subsequent visits have included a brief neurological evaluation to determine if I have gotten worse. So far, I am holding steady.

My vision is my greatest problem. The disease limits my ability to process sight. My eyes see things normally but my brain doesn't process the same signal. This is a huge simplification of the issue, but basically that's the problem. I have issues walking when there is a sidewalk or curb. Gary and I went to breakfast several months ago. I was walking through the parking lot and didn't see the curb. I tripped and fell hard to the ground. My hands and knees were pretty cut up and I still have knee pain. Now when we walk, Gary points out all holes or curbs or any object that I might not see.

Now that I know what is wrong, I can learn to deal with it. I am grateful for my family's understanding and help. Thank goodness for my friend PJ. She keeps me grounded and able to laugh.

EARLY SIGNS—PJ: PJ and her husband, Bob, just before PJ started this book, moved from Florida to Central New York, and both are retired. At present, however, they live in Canada, where Bob has family. PJ has two children from a previous marriage, Char and Tiffany, and four grandchildren. She is very dependent on her daughter, who became her caregiver while she was in Syracuse. She, like Sue, had to wait many months for a diagnosis of early stage Alzheimer's, but is having trouble accepting the changes in her life.

EARLY SIGNS—PJ

Hi – My name is Patricia Joleen Moore Kimmerly, PJ for short, and sometime between 2004 and 2005, at about age 63, I began noticing memory lapses. I had always had a functional habit of keeping copious notes in a Day Minder notebook, then filing away each completed book. This had become a lifelong ritual, and when I started having problems, it was, in retrospect, a harbinger of a definite future need.

About five years ago, I noticed that my adult habit of using the Day Minder was no longer as functional for me. I would forget to write things down. I had gaps and couldn't go back and remember what I was trying to say. It was as if I had some kind of brain injury. My OB/GYN doctor, during an annual exam visit, asked me a couple of simple questions and I couldn't answer them. I couldn't stay in bed and sleep, so I was sleep deprived, as well as under stress, related to marital problems between my husband and me. We even separated for a time. I can't imagine why that happened then because Bob and I now have a strong relationship.

I knew something was wrong, and we even went to lawyers, but I couldn't give a reason why we should get a divorce. We knew Bob's mother probably had Alzheimer's, but he didn't recognize it with me. It was apparently the first signs of the disease. When I shared these concerns with my doc, she recommended neuro-psych testing to rule out "difficulties not visible with MRI and computed axial tomography scans." I've always reacted rather than sitting back waiting for issues to more clearly present themselves, so I was eager to take the tests.

The Truth Will Set You Free

If I didn't have a journal in some form, I was sure I couldn't function. It would be like being in a new country without a map. I function now just by default. I want to stay alive, and I want to do the best I can. But the challenges and reminders are constant that I am not what I used to be. It's harrowing. Sometimes, I can say this is as good as it gets and I'm still a person, and that's okay, but it's not going to stay this way. Then I think about the future and ask myself what can I do then, what do I have to do?

It's just that constant struggle that I feel I have to engage in, but there are no answers. The idea of this book, however, is that it guarantees that we can attain a part of immortality. If our ideas, our words, our thoughts are written somewhere, it validates that we were here. I don't know why that's so important to me, but it is. The label of Alzheimer's or dementia has a negative identity, and most people see us as incapable of communicating. Not so. Not at all.

My Story

Although my days now focus more on worry about what the future has in store, I do have some fun memories of my past. After graduation from college as an English teacher, I was offered a job teaching 7th grade English in Kenosha, Wisconsin, which is the greater-Chicago area. In those days, in the '60s and '70s, students weren't molded into certain ways of thinking and behaving. I was sharing an apartment in a women's residence building with a teacher from the same school. Neither she nor I did much cooking and spent most of our paychecks eating out. One of my students would have pizza delivered.

My first experience trying to cook was getting a piece of frozen meat at the store and putting it on the pilot light on the stove and leaving it there while I was at school. The stench was unbelievable when I got home. After that, Sharon and I decided we would go out as much as possible. My boyfriend from college was still pursuing me at the time, and we continued to date long distance. The following summer we got married—huge mistake. His grandfather was a successful inventor. Honeywell bought his temperature control, and the family had money—for instance, an 85-foot yacht on the St. Lawrence River—but, unfortunately, my husband at the time was a functioning alcoholic, and things just didn't work out. We do have two great children. When we eventually divorced, I became involved with a friend of his, and we married and moved to Ithaca, NY. We made it for about 10 years and we too got divorced. My children had never really trusted him.

I was involved in the Comprehensive Employment and Training Act (CETA) program teaching work skills and creating jobs for young people. I tracked them, encouraged them, and counseled them. It was a government program and eventually the funding was dropped. I decided at some point—I get unclear about the sequence of events—that marriage was something I didn't really do well, and after I got rid of husband #2, I went to graduate school with two kids at home and a full-time job. It was really great but difficult. I earned a master's in rehabilitation. I went to work for a brain injury program as a case manager with about 20 clients. I ultimately moved to Maryland to work at a rehab facility. I stayed until that program ended and moved to New York State, where I was on the faculty at Cornell University. My job was to accommodate people with disabilities in businesses all over the US, Puerto Rico, and the Virgin Islands.

While I was studying at Cornell and before I even gave a thought to memory problems, I gave a talk to 400 medical staff and administrators of Westchester County Medical Association and suddenly heard ringing in my ears. I had no real sense of what I was saying. I just fell apart, yet continued reading my notes. Someone's cell phone was feeding into my microphone and it triggered these symptoms. I had recorded the speech and when playing it again after the presentation I heard myself reciting everything in a monotone. I was so embarrassed. I'll never forget that—the disconnected sense and great fear—but the individual reviews from the participants were surprisingly great.

My third husband, Bob Kimmerly, and I were married in August of 1994. After I married Bob, I quit my job though I hated to do it. We spent summers in the Thousand Islands and winters in Florida. During our first two years together, we rented a condo in Florida. Finally, after having spent several years dividing our time between our New York home on Hill Island on the St. Lawrence River, less than a mile from the Canadian border, and our winter condo in Florida, Bob and I decided to sell our river home and the Duty Free Store my husband owned there and move to Cape Coral, Florida. Florida was grand. I began volunteering at the Alzheimer's facility and even tried golf. Bob is a dedicated golfer. He was on one golf course or another six days a week—and sometimes seven days. I enjoyed being outdoors in winter, but I did not enjoy the highly competitive attitudes of the women's groups and even the couples' groups at the golf clubs. Golf was not for me, although for Bob's sake, I did try.

At the time, I began having noticeable problems. My husband and I were permanent residents of Cape Coral, having bought a house on a lake that connected to several other lakes via canals, eventually flowing to the Gulf of Mexico. Walls of sliding glass doors opened to "our" lake from our large lanai. We were a block from Cape Coral Parkway, which provided a direct route to Fort Myers with one toll bridge. In two words, "our paradise."

Searching for a Diagnosis

At one point, about nine years after my monotone speech at Cornell, my daughter, Tiffany, and her husband, Eric, called on me when they were involved in attending training classes for a new business, and I went up to Oakville, Ontario, to babysit for my two grandchildren in a high-rise overlooking Ontario Lake. My younger grandchild was at an age where she never wanted her parents to leave—and they were spending 8 to 15 hours a day in training. Every time they left, and sometimes they would be in or out during the day, she would cry uncontrollably and nothing would comfort her. In the meantime, I had been asked to tutor her sister, 7 years old, in math. I've had a problem with numbers my entire life. Numbers and I never got along, and when I tell people that, they question how I could have a master's degree. I don't know, but I do have one. I only had to take one basic math course that whole time, and I managed to pass it. In my work, I've always had good secretaries, good accountants, and I hate to admit it, but they did cover for me without comment.

A few years passed, and my forgetfulness increased to a point where I felt I must find out why. When I was first referred to a neurologist-psychologist, Dr. J.T., I was eager to "check and see," since I had concentrated in traumatic brain injury and other neurological impairments for my master's degree in 1986. The results, according to her, were not good, indicating, in her view, severe deficits in processing and logic tests (most of which were math). I told her my math deficits had plagued me since age 8, when I was bedridden with rheumatic fever for an entire year without any home tutoring. She was not impressed, asking how I could have earned a bachelor's degree without math courses, let alone a master's. I offered to show her my CVs, but she refused. I've had other good friends respond the same way. So, Dr. J.T. and I parted ways.

I then started going to a neurologist in Naples, Fla., who treated his patients with vitamin supplementation. He has and sells his own brand of supplements—no conflict, right? Because a close friend and neighbor who believed this doctor kept him alive with vitamins against all odds, I wanted to give it a try. You can only imagine the cost of my vitamin supplementation regimen! It had little effect, and after spending thousands of dollars on vitamins, I gave it up. He did suggest a third option, a psych evaluation, which I had already had with Dr. J.T. and failed miserably. To my great consternation, the doctor he wanted to refer me to was Dr. J.T., the very same doctor who had done the original battery of tests. Later, in the car on our way home, I broke down and sobbed about what was happening to me and asking why my efforts to find answers or help for my increasing symptoms were failing.

Prior to my most recent diagnosis of early stage AD, I felt I had been led down a few "garden paths." In retrospect, I am now certain my lapses in memory and feeling confused were present much earlier than I was willing to admit to myself or others. I didn't feel that I was functioning the way I should—something wasn't right. There was a sense of "offness." Looking back now, if I had been less inhibited, I should have stood up and smacked those doctors in the face. I have since attended an Alzheimer's support group and met my co-author, Sue Dublin.

Because my husband, Dave, had so many physical problems, the last thing the doctors looked at was a diagnosis of Alzheimer's, but when Dave was finally diagnosed, it was less than a year before his death. I've learned so much recently about the disease, I am including my story as a contrast to Early Onset Alzheimer's and Early Stage Alzheimer's.

EARLY SIGNS—DAVE

Although Alzheimer's has certain characteristics that would appear to separate it from other diseases, it might well be connected if a patient has illnesses such as congestive heart failure or cardiovascular disease, where lack of oxygen has caused irreversible damage. My husband had several procedures to open clogged arteries, and each time, it took him longer to regain his ability to reason. When the characteristics of Alzheimer's are also present, a diagnosis of vascular dementia could be a definite possibility. Certain signs that indicate AD also occur in vascular dementia.

What are the characteristics that suggest Alzheimer's? In the early stages, the symptoms are not that noticeable. They could be caused by all kinds of circumstances, for instance, oxygen deprivation. David was diagnosed with congestive heart failure more than 10 years ago. He was a retired teacher and I was a freelance writer. We had been doing a lot of traveling, but following his second cardiac triple-bypass, on one of our cross country trips, he lost memories of his immediate past—vacations, previous cross-country trips, etc.—and never regained them. His ability to lead a normal life, however, did not change at that time.

At age 70 he showed normal signs of aging, although his recurrent bouts with CHF took their toll. He could drive, enjoyed playing cards, especially cribbage, did the laundry, and made the bed every day. We were living in a retirement community, El Dorado Ranch, on the Baja Peninsula in Mexico, 2-1/2 hours south of the US Border. We led an active social life with others in the community. Dave enjoyed water volleyball at the pool, and we were planning to make it our permanent home, traveling to Western Massachusetts for a month or two each year to visit our children and grandchildren.

We celebrated our 50th wedding anniversary in 2007. Dave was 78. We flew to Massachusetts and had a wonderful family reunion with family from both sides. We flew back in September, picked up our car from a friend's house in El Centro, CA, and drove to El Dorado. We were fine until February 2008. Dave was retaining fluids and had difficulty walking and breathing, and Lasix, his prescription drug, wasn't helping. We drove to El Centro and his cardiologist there had him transported to Scripps Green Hospital in San Diego. This was the beginning of Dave's downward spiral.

He was transported again to Scripps Green in July in order to bring his system back to normal. The major problem had to do with his lab work being abnormal as well as fluid retention. It became evident that we would have to return to Massachusetts for good. Trying to keep him on an even keel in Mexico was not working. Even though medical assistance was available, the specialized care he needed was not.

The Changing Face of Dementia

After his July hospital stay, however, he began to show strange symptoms, hallucinating, obsessing about a cut on his arm, using oxygen most of the time, and being up all night, then sleeping most of the day. I did keep a journal during this time and it was obvious he was suffering from some form of dementia, although he still had not been diagnosed with AD. At night he would sit up on the side of the bed with his head in his hands. He was convinced there was someone else in bed with us. Eventually, he actually had a sense of humor about the stranger in bed with us. When he decided he needed something, there was no reasoning with him. For instance, one morning he put on a long-sleeved white shirt while the temperature outside was 115 degrees. He discovered it had yellow spots on it, and he insisted in looking through all his shirts until he found another long-sleeved white shirt without spots.

At this point, Dave was still driving, but it soon became evident that he was having difficulty, and my husband who had always taken great pride in his driving ability—he had been a driver education teacher for many years—turned long-distance driving over to me. He was preoccupied with the injury to his arm after a fall and kept taking the bandage off, which just made it start to bleed again. Every night he would wake me between 3 and 5 a.m. for one reason or another. Thank God for our friend, June Martin. When we had car trouble for a week, she made sure we had enough groceries.

You can't reason with those who have AD to change their minds about an activity they consider necessary. Arguments are useless.

Dave wasn't always accepting of things I asked him to do—eat dinner, take a shower, take medication, etc. That's when he gave me a double identity—"Good Marge" and "Bad Marge." I was Bad Marge when I stopped him from emptying the closet and packing all our clothes long before we planned to leave the area. He was very concerned that he didn't have the energy to do it anyway.

We made plans to go to El Centro for Dave's doctor's appointment in August 2008, then go to San Diego, arrange to have our car shipped, and fly home. It was more complicated than that. Dave was again hospitalized, being transported by helicopter from El Centro. His lungs were full of fluid. He apparently had been taking his medications more than once a day. It was evident that he was experiencing "sundowning," a state of confusion experienced at the end of the day and into the night, a symptom that often occurs in people with dementia, such as Alzheimer's disease. When I was signing David out of the hospital in San Diego in February 2008, the nurse told me that David had less than six months to live. I was in shock. I knew Dave had physical problems, but those could be treated, and I reported the nurse for telling me such a thing. As it turned out, David didn't die in six months; he died a year later.

Our plane trip east after Dave was discharged from the hospital in July 2008 was a nightmare. He had no patience with the vagaries of plane travel. By the time we reached the last leg of our trip, he became stubborn, so much so that he took his pants off and refused to put them back on. He was wearing Depends and wouldn't leave the plane. Finally, EMTs and State Troopers convinced him to cooperate. As soon as he saw our children, Carl and Dena, he calmed right down. However, we took him to Berkshire Medical Center in Pittsfield, and he had to be there for a week. His whole physical system needed stabilizing, and he became violent the first few nights. This was highly unusual behavior for David, who had always had an even disposition, and I was heartbroken at what was happening to him. That's when he was finally diagnosed with AD, and because we were waiting for an apartment at Providence Court, an assisted care facility, he had to go to a nursing home until October 1 while I stayed with my daughter, Dena.

BIBLIOGRAPHY

Croisile, Dr. Bernard. 2004. "Benson's Syndrome or Posterior Cortical Atrophy." *Orphanet Encyclopedia*. http://www.orpha.net/data/patho/GB/uk-Benson.pdf.

Fackelmann, Kathleen. 2007. "Who Thinks of Alzheimer's in Someone So Young?" *USA Today*, Accessed December 6. http://www.usatoday.com/news/health/2007-06-11-alzheimers-cover_N.htm.

Smith, Glenn, PhD. 2011. "Alzheimer's: Sundowning. Mayo Clinic." http://www.mayoclinic.com/health/sundowning/HQ01463.

What Happens When You Are Diagnosed with Alzheimer's Disease?

*D*epending on your age, you may accept your need for assistance, but some people are not at all prepared. When suddenly faced with job loss or dependence on others, they spend months or years waiting for some kind of diagnosis before they finally find a neurologist who is willing to put a name to their symptoms. Sue and PJ share their experiences below, following their diagnosis.

SHARING THE DIAGNOSIS—SUE

Once we ruled out most other options, we told the children about the diagnosis. When we decided to go to Boston, we told them why we were going. Lizzie, our youngest, didn't understand at first, as she didn't know what the disease was. Ben and Kaitie "hit the books" and started reading. They are all very positive about it now. I imagine they have talked together about it but family dinners are just as they used to be, except Gary does most of the cooking. Kaitie organized a group to participate in the Alzheimer's Annual Memory Walk. She raised a lot of money for the cause and got many to contribute.

Because Alzheimer's disease (AD) primarily affects older adults, the younger population faces unique challenges with diagnosis, care, and stigma.

(ALZ.ORG, 2011)

MISUNDERSTANDINGS ABOUT THE DISEASE

When I told Mom about the diagnosis, I was so tense I could hardly pronounce the word "Alzheimer's." Initially, she couldn't believe the diagnosis because she couldn't see any changes in me. She couldn't understand how I could have the disease.

Alzheimer's was—and often still is—a disease no one talked about or acknowledged. Therefore, when it was discussed in the family, it was matter of fact, impersonal, not a disease that I had. Even so, Mom was very supportive, always wanting to know the test results. She may have been in denial because she couldn't grasp how I could have it if I didn't really show the signs and I was so young. Truthfully, we all just went on with our normal lives. When there was a challenge for me, we would either bypass the issue or work through it. Life as usual for the family.

We were really more focused on Mom's issues than mine. I would go on medical appointments with her; I would go over to the house and do dishes. It was more about Mom than me. My mom's health started getting worse, and with her needing care a lot of time, it was probably my hardest time. She had emphysema and I couldn't seem to help her with things for which she needed help. I spent a lot of time over there. We were talking about home care and having somebody come in to help, and she was hallucinating. She was having a problem with that, I guess. She was

30

having a difficult time and I was having difficulty helping her, loading and unloading the dishwasher the way she wanted it. It was again spatial things, and it took a tremendous amount of energy to do that for her; sometimes, she was really upset, and kind of yelled at me, so to speak, which was probably the first time in my life I experienced that, and it was very painful. She had a lot of doctor's appointments, so I went to the appointments with her and helped with things like pushing the wheelchair that she used when she was going to the doctor, and the tech that did the lab work said, "You're all set?" I was trying to maneuver the wheelchair and she said, "I see you have no experience in making these things work," and she gave me a little tutorial, and I thought to myself about how many times I had taken care of patients in wheelchairs.

> The emotion behind failing words is far more important than the words themselves and needs to be validated.
>
> (KOENIG-COSTE, p. 7)

Then Mom started really going downhill, Doug, my brother, was here from Massachusetts wanting to know what was happening, and it was so hard. I couldn't come up with words and terms to be able to explain to the family what the doctors are talking about. Normally, I would be able to do that without difficulty and I just felt so frustrated and shut down that I couldn't even help in my area of expertise. That was very, very hard.

Once I came home and had a diagnosis from Dr. Press of posterior cortical atrophy (PCA), an unusual form of Alzheimer's. I called the Alzheimer's Association to get some information because I really didn't know too much about it. I started making calls and asked if there were any support groups or literature, etc., and I spoke with one of their representatives who said at this time there weren't any groups for people with early onset Alzheimer's. One thing led to another, and he wanted me to talk to another person who worked there who could introduce me to yet another person I might want to meet, because she was in the same boat, although she was older.

This is when PJ and I first met. I remember walking into the room and there she was. She was introduced with a little bit of her story. I was, so to speak, shocked—that might be a little harsh—to find out she has her master's in adult education and rehabilitation and was working with Alzheimer's patients, too, so she kind of knew what was going on. She had also done kind of the same thing as I had done. She and her daughter had called the association looking for some guidance, maybe people to talk to, and that's where we started. Right away, we understood each other and knew what we were feeling. She's full of laughter and that helped. She called me one day after she had tried to volunteer at the association for day care for people with Alzheimer's. She kind of freaked out and said, "I shouldn't have done that. That was too close for comfort," and we talked about that for a long time.

After I had been diagnosed, I started with speaking engagements, and when I talked in public for the first time about Alzheimer's I found I got quite a response when they realized how young I was. I went to a health clinic. It was very interesting, and a lot of people stopped and talked, and, again, the guy from the association introduced me with my symptoms and my age and this kept ka-wowing people, making Alzheimer's something that didn't just affect the elderly. Most people hadn't thought about it. We did a walk for Alzheimer's and fundraising was huge.

> There is far too much emphasis on the label, the name and the symptoms generally associated with the disease, and too little emphasis on the individuals who actually have the disease.
>
> (TAYLOR, 2007, p. 12)

What do you say to people who question what you are doing now that you are not working? Trying to educate people about us in general would be useful if we could set up a group of people who want to learn more about the disease. Some people in my support group don't speak up sometimes—shy or not knowing how to contribute. Being able to talk to people who feel what you are feeling is quite remarkable. It's about the feelings. Alzheimer's support groups could be more helpful. Is it a leadership issue? People in our group are not people who share, and perhaps we need to guide them into discussing the illness. We hope that when they leave they can take something away from it. We have five members but no new ones lately. PJ and I are the only early onset members. The others there don't offer much. One guy in the group speaks up once in a while, usually to tell jokes.

When I first joined the group, I thought it would be good, talking about different topics like Alzheimer's and discussing how to cope, but then some of the staff changed, and it's basically pizza every time and chitty-chat. There are frustrations like not being able to drive and that sort of thing that affects everybody in the group. Sometimes caregivers attend the meeting, but most of the time it is just those with the disease.

We've been going to the meetings, but we don't feel we're getting much out of it. We do have a social worker who is willing to work with us to set up our own group in the community.

Once a diagnosis of Alzheimer's has been made, it should be shared with family and friends. In PJ's case, her brother, Bill, was diagnosed with cancer, and PJ was trying to be there for him. When she was finally diagnosed with Alzheimer's, Bill's imminent death was just one more thing to deal with, and, for her, severe depression was the result.

SHARING THE DIAGNOSIS—PJ

After Bob contacted his son-in-law, who set up an appointment with yet another neurologist, I was finally told I had early stage Alzheimer's and was put on Aricept. It was truly a devastating diagnosis. In Florida, my brother, who was five years younger, was very supportive. He had been diagnosed with liver cancer, and we had to support each other. We also had a good friend, Doria, who was there for both of us. Unfortunately, my brother went back to Virginia, where he died much too soon.

I was so alone. I would just sit and stare. That was a clinical sign that I was "going away." When I bought a new coffee pot, you'd think I was buying a washing machine. It was two days before I could plug it in, and it wasn't complicated. It was just put the basket on, put in the coffee and the water in the reservoir, but I was at that point where everything was confusing. I was totally disconnected and my daughter picked up on it. She packed up her two kids and came down to Florida to see for herself what was going on with me. I knew something was really wrong, and I knew I needed help. Trying to figure it out was like writing my own obituary. I didn't know what was going on, and I didn't know how to defend myself against it. I was terrified. There was that constant switching between what was my reality and what I wanted to be my reality. I tried to be positive, but I cried a lot. I couldn't sleep at night; couldn't stay asleep for two hours at a time. I tried to rationalize, to realize that it wasn't my fault; I didn't cause these things to happen. It frustrated me and it angered me, and I didn't know how to sort those emotions out. And Bob was golfing. I was glad he was golfing and I knew he needed it, but I resented that he could enjoy something and come home and take a nap. I was trying to deal with my feelings, and I felt I should be able to do that, to the point of obsessing.

In regards to driving, the doctor had to report to the state my symptoms and my diagnosis. I took the test and I passed it, but that didn't matter. Even after passing the tests—practical, written, and vision—the ball was dropped and too much time passed. I missed the "paper" deadline and my license was revoked. That was devastating.

My daughter, Tiffany, has been with me a hundred percent and it was she who talked me into contacting the Alzheimer's Association and meeting Sue after Bob and I moved to Central New York to be close to Tiffany. I think I'm doing pretty well. I'm not crying all the time. I haven't hurt anyone, or killed anyone.

I never trusted my memory. I have always depended on my Day Minder. If I didn't have a journal in some form, I was sure I couldn't function. It would be like being in a new country without a map. I function now just by default. I want to stay alive, and I want to do the best I can. But the challenges and reminders are constant that I am not what I used to be. It's harrowing.

BEING A CAREGIVER WHILE NEEDING ONE

With Alzheimer's, the needs of family members sometimes lead to the need for caregiving before AD has been diagnosed. Sue found herself responsible for her mother's care, and my brother, Roger Willis "Bill" Moore, endured several months with me when I was having cognitive problems but had not yet been diagnosed with AD.

Bill had moved from California to Punta Gorda, Florida, a 30 to 45 minute trip from our home in Cape Coral, and purchased a live-on-board sailboat. That this sailboat soon revealed itself as non-seaworthy was the first in a cluster of bad decisions on his part. He supported himself by earning a commercial boat captain's license and operated a variety of cruises and private fishing expeditions in the Gulf.

Bill joined an online dating/matchup service. The woman with whom he developed a relationship couldn't have been more wrong for him. In a nutshell, Bill began spending more than he could ever make. In a short time, he was instructing my husband not to take any calls that might be for him. He was spending money he didn't have and creditors hunted him. This quickly became a real imposition for us. We were getting upwards of 20 collection calls for him each day. Even caller ID became useless, as the collectors became cleverer. This was only the beginning of Bill's downward spiral.

As a Vietnam veteran, he regularly went to the VA Hospital in St. Pete, Florida, for his health care. One morning, friends of my brother at the marina called me to ask if Bill was with us. They had not seen him in two days, though his dog, Chesty Puller—named for a legendary Marine, was aboard the boat.

They were worried. Bob and I immediately drove to the marina. I went aboard with great trepidation—and found my brother comatose with Chesty keeping guard over him. I could not elicit any response from him other than a pulse. I dashed off the boat and called 911. The ambulance arrived shortly. The efforts to remove a 6'2" grossly overweight comatose man from a lower berth was a huge undertaking. I rode in the ambulance and my husband followed. Bill was diagnosed with Toxic Liver Disease soon after he was admitted to the St. Pete VA Hospital. Weeks passed, and Bob and I visited him regularly; his son, Jason, flew in from California (Jason, at that time, was Paris Hilton's PR agent.) Bill couldn't help telling everyone about his conversation with Paris when she called him.

After six weeks, the good folks at the VA hospital decided to go for broke and send him to the VA hospital in Richmond, Virginia, to be evaluated for a liver transplant. The only catch was that someone must be with him during the entire evaluation period. I was the only viable candidate. We were flown with a medic corporate jet to Richmond. The VA social worker arranged housing for me in "a VA hotel."

Dory was my initial VA transporter. She immediately became my friend, support person, and "caretaker." I was lonely, afraid, confused, and often the recipient of my brother's fearful anger. Dory would transport me to and from the hospital and the family residence, even on her days off. I had my meals in the VA cafeteria, and Dory would often join me. Most of my fellow residents kept food in the residents' kitchen and several cooked daily. With few exceptions, these individuals were so exhausted from spending time with their loved ones, they could not summon the energy to socialize. I was so lonely.

A diagnosis of Alzheimer's in Dave's case was not surprising given the symptoms he showed, but if it had been made sooner, accepting it would have been easier for both of us.

ACCEPTING THE DIAGNOSIS—DAVE

We were fortunate in being able to move into an apartment in an assisted living building in October 2008 after he was diagnosed. That meant Dave was able to meet with a nurse inside the building to have his blood pressure checked. By the time we were settled into our apartment, he was using portable oxygen most of the time and used a walker to get around. He continued to be up at night and sleep most of the day. I did try to keep him as active as I could. He didn't have much appetite, but I tried to make sure there were snacks that he liked. He began to see a neurologist, Dr. Jay Ellis, whom I knew from when I worked at the hospital in Pittsfield 20 years earlier. He tried to set Dave up in a clinical trial, but it didn't work out because one of Dave's medicines negated his eligibility.

We did play cards with other residents and that was fun, but Dave ultimately stopped going when he wasn't winning enough to suit him. Also, he stopped taking showers, and the one time I managed to convince him to take a bath instead, he wasn't able to get out of the tub and he was too heavy for me. I had to call our son Carl to help me. No more baths. I had always depended on Dave to do dishes, make the bed, and do laundry. He was always so helpful, but he stopped doing dishes and making the bed. He continued to do the laundry until the time I received a call from one of the tenants who told me Dave had opened the door on every drier and didn't close any of the doors, so that other people doing their laundry returned to find wet clothes. No more laundry. Sometimes, he would go down the elevator to the first floor to buy a soda, and after a while, when he didn't come back, I would go down to find him. It seems he had forgotten to buy the soda and forgotten to come back to the apartment. He was sitting in the dining hall waiting for someone to come and get him.

Dave had trouble with balance and a couple of times fell in the hall, one time because his walker broke when he was leaning too hard on it. I had to call 911 for the firemen to come and help him get up. We managed pretty well through Christmas and into the new year, 2009. After a few weeks, however, he started to go downhill.

Life with Dave was a 24-7 caregiving situation, but I wouldn't have traded it for anything. For a while, he kept driving in town, but his neurologist, Dr. Ellis, managed to convince him to give up driving, for which I breathed a sigh of relief. His memory was slowly getting worse and he had trouble knowing if it was morning or night, when he was supposed to take his medications, where we were living, and was amazed that I knew where to go when we went out in the car. Sometimes he would ask me if I was his wife, and other times he would apologize for being such a nuisance.

Unfortunately, in March, Dave was again hospitalized. Even though I had tried to hide his medications, I do think he would find them while he was wandering in the night and take several at once. In addition to congestive heart failure (CHF), Dave had peripheral artery disease, and even when using a walker had trouble ambulating. He was very apt to fall, and I couldn't get him up. He also had prostate cancer and newly diagnosed diabetes. While in the hospital, he was catheterized because the staff couldn't keep up with his lack of continence. The catheter was not the right size and caused bleeding, which compounded his problems.

Finally, on March 5 he was discharged from the hospital, and on the morning of March 6, 2009, he died peacefully in bed at home. He was a good, loving man, well-liked by everyone who knew him, and our life together was more fun than sorrow. My only regret is that I didn't know then what I know now about Alzheimer's. I would have understood his symptoms so much better. Our life together in those final days could have been more relaxed.

It's been over three years since Dave died, and I miss him terribly, but I still have the memories before Alzheimer's and, just as important, during Alzheimer's. The one thing we both had in all our time together, 52 years, was a sense of humor. It was so much easier to accept with humor the difficulties that faced us. Early in our marriage, Dave used to tell people who hadn't met me yet that I was impossible to live with, and when they met me, they would say, "Gosh, Dave, she isn't bad at all. She's really nice." I always wondered if they would say that if he hadn't set them up. Another little joke of his was that his mother made him and his siblings take a bath every day—and once a week, she changed the water. This sense of humor carried over into our immediate family, and family get-togethers have always been and are still a time of great laughter. Even when he had Alzheimer's, he never lost his sense of fun. When the doctor or nurse would ask him the questions they always ask—"How old are you?", "What year is it?"—he would deliberately give the wrong answer, grin from ear to ear, and then tell them what they wanted to hear. Probably the easiest time he had with the disease is when he temporarily had to go to a nursing home for a couple of months. At the time, I was staying with my daughter, her daughter and husband, and twin boys two years old. We couldn't move into senior housing until October and the nursing home was the only option. At first, he didn't really understand where he was, but he quickly made friends with the staff and they treated him with great love and care, so much so that after we did move into our apartment, he twice wanted to go back to Hillcrest Commons to see his friends. They were so pleased to see him and he was equally pleased to see them. In the nursing home, he carried his wallet everywhere and was extremely upset if he couldn't find it. Once, we found it in the wastebasket in the bathroom.

BIBLIOGRAPHY

Koenig-Coste, Joanne. 2004. *Learning to Speak Alzheimer's*. Boston: Mariner Books.

4

Coping from Day to Day

*A serious difficulty faced by someone with Alzheimer's
disease (AD) is the sense of being all alone, which
ultimately leads to depression. Far too many people lack
knowledge about AD and tend to avoid people who have it.
Also, support groups so far do not encourage people with
early stage or early onset Alzheimer's to create their own
group and share with each other.*

LIVING WITH ALZHEIMER'S—SUE

At my daughter Kait's wedding, thinking I was asking a close
friend, "Dick," to dance, I went up to him and said, "I've been
looking for you all night for a dance." The problem was that it
wasn't Dick. Truth is, I tried that twice. Neither was Dick. So I
gave up. Never did dance with Dick. Four high school friends
came to the wedding, and I was apprehensive, as I hadn't seen
some of them in a long time. I was concerned how they would
react to me. However, we had a wonderful time together—lots of

laughs. They helped me when I needed it. There's nothing like old friends. My thanks to Susan, Anne, Lindsay, and Gail.

Another time, when Gary was out of town, an old friend called to confirm our lunch date for that day. All of my safety nets were gone. I didn't have clothes ready or anything. I wanted to cancel, but decided to go. I chose clothing that I knew I had worn before. It took a long time to get dressed, making sure things were on correctly. I was anxious I wouldn't be ready on time, looking out the window for Nena to come. I watch cable TV because the time is on the screen. I was ready two or three hours early and paced until Nena came. When the doorbell rang, I gave myself a high 5. I did it, and we had a great time. PJ and I talked about these time issues. We both spend a lot of time waiting—we don't want to be late. We have such a need to be *on time*. It has changed for us. We are concerned that we will forget what we have to do and miss an appointment or a luncheon date. I do have a problem with my vision, which was okay two and half years ago. Not now. It's the type of Alzheimer's I have. It adversely affects vision.

I watch cable TV because the time is on the screen.

SUE

At home, Gary is my savior. I can't do puzzles or crafts anymore, but Gary keeps me challenged on a daily basis. I try to put my shoes on, try to tie them, empty the dishwasher, feed the dogs, set the table, and other household chores. Some days are better than others. Sometimes, it takes hours to do one thing, but Gary accepts that and keeps encouraging me. He lets me think through a task, ask questions. We also walk often, many times per week. Sometimes we just walk around the neighborhood; other times, we visit the farmer's market, craft shows, antique shows, and even the grocery store. We both feel exercising brain and body is very necessary.

UNDERSTANDING ALZHEIMER'S—PJ

I'm having what I refer to as my "random neuron firing." My thoughts are coming so fast, so disjointed, so irrelevant to this moment, I can't even record them. "Why?" I keep silently asking. I can feel my thoughts scrambling for some kind of order—some kind of revelation or missed bit of clarity. I've had this sense more frequently the last few days. I can't see or feel the cause. Sometimes I feel as though the answer to what fuels these episodes is just on the tip of my brain's tongue ... my gosh, I hate this. It's like watching *Jeopardy*—I'm so close to the answer, yet the correct answer is playing a hide and seek game, a game with weird rules.

Where do these thoughts come from? Who puts the scramble in my memory? These episodes scare me, provoking fear that the guarding barricades surrounding what's left of my thinking mind are getting weaker by the day.

One problem I have in my daily routine is choosing what I'm going to wear and remembering what I wore yesterday. I've tried to devise a system, and when I've worn something, I put it into one of those sorters on wheels where you put whites and colors. I pay a lot of attention to this because when I was working, I was overly organized, and regardless of Alzheimer's, that's who I am. What disturbed me the most after testing was trying to talk to people who said they too had memory problems all the time, acting as if I was not telling the truth when I told them I had AD. People are so relieved that they don't have our symptoms. "How do you know you have it?" It's like living in a different country and not being able to speak the language.

I struggle with my Day Minder. Sometimes I start with it and think, "Oh, for heaven's sake, why am I doing this?" I think it's my insecurity thing. If I don't try it, I won't mess it up and embarrass myself. I need to get over that and do a better job of it. The problem is I have to be more consistent with what kind of material I write it on so I can retrieve it. It's an organizational problem.

In reading the previous paragraphs, I'm afraid I'm becoming the overly-dramatic "nut job." I miss my mental downtimes when studying for a class or prepping a training exercise for a group to whom I was providing mandated information for compliance with new federal and state laws and practices. Today was the day, as noted, of "random neuron firing." I could not get into a stride, a connection, if you will, with my world. I feel disconnected, valueless, unwanted, unneeded, totally irrelevant. How long will this sense—or non-sense—be in the forefront of my mind (or whatever is instructing my thoughts). This feeling is exhausting, demeaning, terrifying. I can certainly see why suicide might enter the thoughts of someone diagnosed with Alzheimer's.

UNDERSTANDING ALZHEIMER'S—DAVE

When Dave and I moved into our assisted living apartment, close to family and friends, in October of 2008, I was anxious to get him involved in the activities available at the Senior Center. It was also a way for me to have some time to myself. Because of his trouble walking and need for a walker and oxygen, it was difficult to get him down the elevator, out the door to the car, and to the Senior Center about a half-mile drive away. He cooperated, but not too willingly.

The way the program was set up was to introduce ourselves around the room, have sandwiches and a drink, and allow those with AD to leave for activities while we, the caregivers, discussed the problems we were facing on a daily basis. I had hoped Dave could be active in wood shop, but it wasn't available during the time we were there. Bingo was, however, and he was taken there. He hated Bingo. His way of dealing with a situation he didn't like was to get stubborn and refuse to participate. When I took him home, he was pretty annoyed with everything. He said he wasn't going to attend anymore. Between convincing him to return to the Senior Center and going to doctor's appointments on a regular basis, he started going downhill. He didn't want to leave the apartment, didn't want to eat, refused to shower, needed help getting dressed, and wore Depends all the time, day and night. Every once in awhile, he would ask me if I was his wife.

As it turned out, he only went one more time to the Senior Center, and with the help of the staff, we were setting up a program for him to attend day care about three times a week and participate in activities he enjoyed. Unfortunately, Dave was admitted to the hospital in March 2009 and never did go to the Senior Center again.

———————

According to Sue and PJ's experiences at support group meetings, they have been able to contribute to the group, even though they were the only ones in the early stages of AD. It is difficult for people involved in public support programs to encourage those with beginning or early onset AD, for one reason because it sometimes takes so long to receive a diagnosis, for another reason because those who have been diagnosed have trouble accepting the diagnosis. In addition, the economy has caused a decrease in funds, and layoffs have created a shortage of social workers who are willing or able to create a group more geared to early stage patients. The group Sue and PJ attended and the group I attended both focused on the caregiver.

Recently, I read a 2010 article by Alan Dienstag about encouraging Alzheimer's patients to participate in a writing workshop. What they offered was anything from sheer poetry to material that was difficult to read, but revealing, nonetheless. It is important to get as many contributions as we can from people who have the disease. Sue and PJ have made it clear in this book that they have a lot to say in writing, even though they have trouble articulating their feelings out loud to others.

ADDING TO QUALITY OF LIFE

An important aspect of treating Alzheimer's is finding a way to keep the person involved and interested. Dienstag listed several challenges for members of support groups who have the disease and those caring for them. Therapy for Alzheimer's patients and their families includes presenting outlets such as painting and music, especially music. It offers a way to help express feelings and improve quality of life, as evidenced by an article in *HealthDay.com* by Alan Mozes about a chorus in New York City called "The Unforgettables," comprised of 22 men and women, 11 diagnosed with dementia linked to Alzheimer's disease and 11 caregivers—a spouse, child, or friend. The challenge is to construct a life in the shadow of an advancing disease. Music is a way to connect as evidenced by the joy someone with Alzheimer's exhibits when listening to music or making music. Observing a patient with dementia who is unable to complete a task and then seeing them function in a chorus, singing words and melody, is miraculous.

> "There's a certain camaraderie," noted Howard Smith, a choral member who cares for his wife, Lois, diagnosed with Alzheimer's about two years ago. "Lois is there with people with the same problems. And it's comforting for her [and for all] because it means we're not alone."
>
> (MOZES, 2011)

My husband and I were involved for many years in barbershop choruses, and when Dave was in the nursing home, a member stopped to see him and gave him several CDs of barbershop quartets and choruses. There was little to endear him to nursing home life, but that gift was greatly appreciated. Scott Learn of *The Oregonian* notes that, "research centers increasingly back up the insight that the brain's musical pathways remain intact longer, even after speech and short-term memory fade." This was evident when country singer Glenn Campbell announced that he had Alzheimer's, and then performed some of his greatest hits without a hitch at the 2012 Grammys. A hint of his illness was present when he finished singing and asked someone where he should go now.

If a writing workshop is formed, participants are encouraged to write about things they remember. The act of remembering is not lost for those with the disease, and writing down memories is a way to validate self. This book is exactly that for Sue and PJ, and they are well aware of it. If you re-read what you've written, you may not remember having written it, but there it is, a "confirmation of self."

In addition to music and writing projects, theater and art are also used as vehicles to keep those with AD active and involved. A seven-week session of improve theater called the Memory Ensemble was instituted by the Feinberg School of Medicine at Northwestern University and the Looking Glass Theater Company. Patients and their caregivers are encouraged to show different emotions by using body language and colors to depict the way they feel.

As noted by Chris Aliades, creativity allows a person with AD or other dementias to express their feelings when words fail. They feel connected and less alone. Art therapy is beneficial as a new way to communicate as well as a way to concentrate. It further has a calming effect on someone with AD. According to Alzheimer's Reading Room, when Lester Potts began painting with watercolors as a visual tool after being diagnosed with AD, he moved from intricate and detailed paintings to more emphasis on color, and, eventually, as the disease progressed, simplistic scenes that reflected peace and a certain acceptance of the life dealt to him.

BIBLIOGRAPHY

Aliades, Chris, MD, January 14, 2009. "Easing Alzheimer's Symptoms With Art Therapy." Medically reviewed by Pat F. Bass III, MD, MS, MPH. Published on EverydayHealth.com. Updated January 14, 2009.

DeMarco, Bob, June 2011 Alzheimer's Reading Room. "An Artist Matures, Painting in Twilight." http://www.alzheimersread ingroom.com/2011/01/art-therapy-and-life-of-alzheimers. html.

Dienstag, Alan, 2010. "Lessons from the Lifelines Writing Group for People in the Early Stages of Alzheimer's Disease: Forgetting What We Don't Remember." *Public Radio*, [Link] http://being. publicradio.org/programs/2010/alzheimers/essay_dienstag-lessonsfromthelifelines.shtml.

Learn, Scott, 2012. "Oregon brothers find music can break through solitude of Alzheimer's disease." *The Oregonian*. Accessed February 7. http://www.oregonlive.com/pacific-northwest-news/index.ssf/2012/02/oregon_brothers_find_music_can. html.

Mozes, Alan, 2011. "Chorus Gives Voice to Those With Alzheimer's." *Health Day*, http://consumer.healthday.com/Article. asp?AID=660103.

5

Making Practical Decisions

*T*he *Alzheimer's Association online tries to keep the public up to date by publishing the latest ways in which those who are faced with Alzheimer's (patients, families, and friends) can create a lifestyle allowing them to deal with the disease until a way is found to treat it. From the national web site, it is possible to enter community web sites. Most of the articles, however, are not written from the viewpoint of the person with the disease. They are written about them. People with Alzheimer's want to make their own decisions when they can, and have been looking at new ways to interact with family and friends.*

PUBLIC PERCEPTION—SUE

As far as support groups go, we have been going to the meetings, but we don't feel we're getting much out of it. We also have decided—and we had a social worker who was willing to work with us—to set up our own group in the community. My problem is writing things down. My vision is deteriorating because of the disease. That's a problem for me, and PJ is very good about writing things down. Sometimes I'll have a good thought. She'll write it down, and then, for me, it's gone.

I am trying to make it through each day without getting too discouraged. I am involved in a monthly book club. Sometimes Gary reads the book to me, and other times, I try to read, but it is difficult and takes a lot of time because of my poor vision. Book club meetings include wine and cheese, usually desserts, snacks, or whatever someone wants to bring. Although they take the book part seriously, it is also a social gathering. There are a few of the members that live nearby and they often ask to drive me to the meeting. Other friends take me on walks, shopping trips, and to lunch. I am so lucky to have close friends who accept me as I am.

In the doctor's office, there is a need for updated information on different kinds of dementia leading to AD. One thing we thought we'd like to do is start a speaker's bureau since we haven't had any requests to speak lately. We talked about this to a social worker and would like to include professionals in a bureau instead of just two people with Alzheimer's. Also, we think home health aides should be educated about how to communicate with their AD patients. If we can form a group, we can put together information for doctors and neurologists to be available in their offices. There is nothing at present that addresses the problems we face with early onset AD. There were pamphlets and information on other neurological diseases but nothing on Alzheimer's. I think that is something we are going to pursue. My general practitioner always asks how things are going and if I need anything. I think overall she definitely focuses on the disease; not for a long time, but enough to acknowledge it.

Gary helps me dress and shower every day, and someone, Gary or our children, helps fix meals. I am no longer independent, but I am so fortunate to have a family who is there for me. I can be alone for several hours, but eventually I become concerned. Marge, PJ, and I have been working on this book for over a year and during that time, our son, Ben, was married, and they now have a baby, Abbie, who visits often. Kaitie was also married last year and we just found out she is pregnant as well.

PUBLIC PERCEPTION—PJ

If you can't *see* it, it doesn't *exist*. This is the way most people perceive AD. If we appear normal and manage to handle social relationships without too much difficulty, many people dismiss the fact that we have this illness called Alzheimer's disease. We don't appear to be sick. Having AD has a huge impact on going out and about, handling physical challenges (stairs), and compensatory actions due to visual difficulties. It is difficult to communicate our thoughts to anyone—and we do have thoughts about how this disease impacts us and how the public perceives us.

Both Sue and I sometimes feel less competent. We so want to hold on to our dignity. We used to do *everything* and now can't do so many things. The attitude of far too many people is that "If you really wanted to do it, you could," and that is so untrue. I waste more time just trying to figure out who and what I am or what I need to do, then berate myself because of these unrealistic concerns about a situation I cannot control.

The two of us try to laugh when we're together about our reaction to the "world around us" and the world's reaction to us (our deficits). When I tell someone I have memory problems, many folks say, "Oh, I do too." They really don't get it. I am very unhappy, not content to have "the disease." We want people to understand the frustration of not "getting it right." It's got nothing to do with effort; I can't always do it. "Just take your time and think." People have no idea what that concept means to us because we functioned very well in real life and communication skills were excellent. Not being able to recall those skills is probably the most frustrating thing about this illness.

A lot needs to be done with the medical profession. They're the ones people trust, and if they lack knowledge about AD, we're the ones who suffer.

PJ

More recently, I am realizing the deterioration has become more real. Like watching yourself go downhill. Like having sunburn and waiting to peel. We should be able to cope better but when we can't, it is difficult. You can ask people with the disease what they are assimilating, but some people just can't articulate. In describing a week or month before a meeting, there is a disconnect that I can feel. I want professionals to tell me how to cope, but do they actually know how to share their knowledge about the disease? They are supposed to be the experts. My voice doesn't mean as much because I have the disease. People are being paid to share their knowledge and can't seem to do it. The powers that be at the Alzheimer's group don't seem to advance. One thing leads to another and it frustrates me because there seems to be a lack of interest.

Reading was my outlet, and now when I read it takes longer and I have to keep going back. I have a basic insecurity going back to childhood; humiliation and embarrassment when trying to communicate now and not being able to explain what I mean. Nobody gets it that we're in a hurry. We don't know how long we're going to be able to do this. A lot *needs* to be done with the medical profession. They're the ones people trust, and if they lack knowledge about AD, we're the ones who suffer.

The present statistics regarding the number of people with AD are cause for concern, but they are possibly already out of date. As baby boomers move into their fifties, there will be more and more people in the early stages of AD, and because so many physicians are hesitant to diagnose early AD, the statistics will continue to be incomplete. The grandchildren of today will become the patients of tomorrow. Fortunately, information about this disease is on the rise, and a recent report published by Alzheimers.org specifically addresses early onset. The information that was not available in the March report is addressed in the new report. The numbers of people with early onset have more than doubled since the first report, and the fact that the Alzheimer's Organization has considered early onset AD a subject for public scrutiny offers hope for the future of those in the early stages of the disease.

Finding out about the disease from the person who has it is the best way to offer insight. Sue Dublin has been involved in giving talks in the community about what is happening to her and how she is coping. PJ and her daughter, Tiffany, were interviewed in an article appearing in the Syracuse *Post Standard*. Both want very much to help people understand this illness better, and as long as they are able to talk about their experiences and encourage others to do so in support groups by tapping into creativity, the public will become more educated about Alzheimer's.

DECISION MAKING

Should a person be told by a primary care physician that he or she has Alzheimer's disease? There are conflicting feelings about the decision. According to G. Richard Holt, primary care physicians when best prepared "will be able to make the appropriate diagnosis and, in a timely manner, inform the patient so that crises can be avoided . . . and the patient can be adequately informed so that choices can be made for the future while decision-making capability remains." Holt also cites, however, a body of opinion against telling the patient because of the stigmatism presently attached to the disease, as well as increased risk of suicide and the possibility of misdiagnosis.

Those who have early stage AD and have accepted the diagnosis want more than anything to be treated with respect. Patience is key when talking with someone who has AD. As Sue and PJ have noted more than once, they are finding that an inordinate amount of time is apt to pass while they are organizing or trying to organize what they want to communicate. The future is not really something they want to face and therefore using up energy to discuss it is not a priority with them. According to Stephen Post of Johns Hopkin University Press, "Keeping the balance is not always easy. Considerations, such as family relationships, the number and availability of caregivers, legal, cultural, religious and financial factors, influence the decision-making process."

The extent to which a person with AD can make simple decisions depends on personality and/or progression of the disease. When a caregiver decides the patient is unable to offer suggestions but does not give the person an opportunity to contribute thoughts on ways to deal with the disease, even though it might take some time, the patient is apt to retreat and not even try. When this happens, it is very possible that some caregivers might put their own interests first.

According to Peter Berger, an editor at *Alzheimer's Weekly*, decision-making is an important part of a person's life, and for those with AD, having caregivers recognize their abilities, even though they might be impaired to a degree, is necessary to maintain confidence and especially self-esteem. For people who have been diagnosed with AD, making decisions on their own eventually leads to giving up control when they are not able to assimilate information that will affect their futures. At that time, it is difficult for them to have a practical conversation about what they might face if no cure is found. Like it or not, they will gradually lose decision-making skills, with longer intervals between being asked questions and being able to answer them. Should a person be told that he or she has AD? Both Sue and PJ were told while they could still make decisions and their reaction was to immediately learn everything they could about the disease before they lost their ability to communicate.

Feelings and emotions remain intact long after words have lost their meaning.

(POST, p. 3)

Because it is difficult to make decisions on another person's behalf, it is important to exhibit patience and understanding, which will lead to an acceptable decision for everyone involved, including the person living with AD. Also, while the individual is still able to contribute to decisions on a daily basis, a plan should be set up for the future, one that will be agreeable to all. Part of these future plans has to do with creating a daily routine that is flexible, changing as needed when the person moves into another phase of the disease.

As AD progresses, instead of offering the patient a complex number of choices, it is better to simplify questions with no more than two choices at a time, for instance, "Would you like hot chocolate or coffee?" If the patient has trouble articulating a choice, he or she might show by facial expression what choice is being made.

In an article by Peter Berger investigating how a husband and wife make decisions, it is noted that "having dementia doesn't mean you automatically lose your decision-making ability—this needs to be considered on a decision-by-decision basis." In addition, "Because dementia is still quite a stigmatized illness, those living with the condition are sensitive to other people's reaction to them. Their confidence can be quite fragile."

ESTABLISHING A NEW ROUTINE

Sue and PJ have had to accept the difficulties that Alzheimer's brings and their ability to communicate their thoughts as time goes on is quite remarkable.

SUE IN JANUARY 2012

Gary is typing this as I can't see the keys nor do I know how to type any longer. It's now January 2012 and my abilities fluctuate day to day. When I sleep well, I seem to be able to get along better during the day than when I have a bad night. Sometimes I'm having trouble brushing my teeth. I don't know why but I can't seem to find the drawer where my toothbrush is. Other days I have no problem at all. I need help with my pills. Gary puts them in a daily pill box but I still can't get the right day. He helps me shower, dress, and makes all our meals. It seems to be pretty normal except when he's not here. I have trouble eating, too. I drop things in my lap and make a mess of the table. The truth is I can't see the food on the plate and don't even know I made a mess. The doctor explains my vision as like trying to see through a straw.

Last night, I went to book club. Barb came and picked me up, helped me get to the car, hooked my seat belt, walked me arm in arm into the house, and carried the wine. I get so frustrated when I'm trying to talk. I know what I want to say, but I usually can't find the words. It's particularly upsetting at the book club or when there are a lot of people around. They all try to be patient with me while I try to tell my story, but it's probably hard for them to wait for my story to come out. Often, I forget what I started to say, and by the time I remember, too much time has passed and I say, "never mind" and we move on. Libraries have "book club" kits for many books. They have several copies and you can reserve them for your group. Dixie got me a copy on CD of this month's book. I can't use the computer but I can listen to the book on the computer. I'm really excited to try and participate in next month's meeting.

The doctor explains my vision as like trying to see through a straw.

Barb also invites me to walk the canal with her. We've had such a gentle winter that we walked a couple of times before the snow came. I'll probably stick to mall walking now until spring. Gary and I play a game where he finishes my sentences when I get stuck. If he guesses right, I say "yes" and if he guesses wrong I say "no." It speeds up our conversations.

Tonight, we are sitting at home waiting to hear from our daughter Lizzie. She has been in El Salvador for a week with Young Life and she comes back to the U.S. tonight. We're watching the flight status report on the Internet. She has gone there five or six times and she loves it.

The snow has finally arrived in Syracuse. We usually are one of the snowiest cities in the United States, but this year we have had very little snow. I think I heard we're something like 80 inches behind last year. The snow provides more challenges for me. I'm not really sure-footed when it's dry, but I'm really having trouble walking in the snow. It's probably because everything is white and everything looks the same to me. I can't see slopes or curbs or anything covered with snow. Putting the dogs out also creates a problem. I have trouble opening and closing the sliding door. I can usually get it opened but sometimes have trouble closing it. It gets cold really fast and someone usually comes to find out why the house is so cold. Our dogs, Rosie and Cassie, give me the uplift I need when I feel down. It's amazing how they can turn a frown into a smile by putting their heads on my lap or kissing my hand or cheek. They really help me almost every day in some way.

I had my six-month check-up with Dr. Press in December. He said things seem pretty good. I've been almost five years into this and I guess I'm doing better than most. I know some of it is the way Gary challenges me. He gently pushes me to make the right decision and challenges my wrong decisions. Sometimes it makes me mad, but I truly think it helps. It certainly keeps me thinking, which is what I should be doing.

I really enjoy when Ben and Lesley bring their daughter Abbie over to visit. It's amazing how quickly she is growing up and developing her personality. I hold her and talk to her as much as I can, but I'm usually fighting for face time with Gary. Kaitie has announced she is going to add to the family too. Brian and Kait are so excited to have a baby, expected in June 2012.

I don't see PJ anymore. She and Bob are in Florida for the winter and go north to Canada for the summer. We talk occasionally on the phone, but not as often as I would like. PJ is the only one I can talk to about certain parts of our disease. She understands the loneliness, the frustration when no one understands me, the feelings, the anger, the peace. Peace may be a strange word, but I truly experience peace. I've always been a calm person; now, not too much bothers me. It's a nice place to be.

Gary and I are going to the Alzheimer's group meeting next Wednesday. They have a monthly meeting for family and patients. They get pizza and everyone sits and talks. We went for a bit two years ago but stopped after five or six meetings. We're going to give it another try. There didn't used to be any direction in the meetings. Basically, everyone just told how they were feeling. I didn't feel as if I was getting anything from the meeting and didn't feel as if I was adding anything positive so I stopped going. I'm looking forward to next week's meeting to see if things have changed at all.

We were trying to decide whether to move into a one-story home or to make changes to our current home. We looked at many new homes but always seemed to be most comfortable with our own home. We recently made some changes so I could be all on one floor. We had the bathroom redone with a large shower and handrails all over and a seat. We moved into a bedroom on that floor too. Basically, we have a patio home that happens to have three floors. We couldn't give up our backyard, especially with grandchildren. So far, this is working great. It's really fun to remodel a house to fit your needs at the time.

I feel things are going as well as can be expected. I can't say enough about the support I get from family and friends.

BIBLIOGRAPHY

Alzheimer's Association. 2010. "Early Onset Dementia: A National Challenge, a Future Crisis." Accessed September 2010. http//www.alz.org/national/documents/report_earlyonset_summary.pdf

Berger, Peter, ed. 2011. "Good Decisions by People with Dementia." *Alzheimer's Weekly,* October 16, 2011.

Post, Stephen. 2000. *The Moral Challenge of Alzheimer's Disease. Ethical Issues from Diagnosis to Dying.* 2nd ed. The Johns Hopkin University Press. http://alzheimer.ca/english/care/ethics-decision.htm

Smith, Amber. 2010. "A Family Faces Alzheimer's Disease; Central New York Mother and Daughter become Patient and Caregiver." *The Post Standard.* September 21.

"What is Alzheimer's?" alz.org 2012. http://www.alz.org/alzheimers_disease_what_is_alzheimers.asp

6

The Role of Caregivers

*L*iving with Alzheimer's is difficult for the person who has
the disease, but equally difficult is the role of caregiver,
especially caring for someone much too young to have such
a disease. Below are comments from family members on how
they have been affected by Alzheimer's disease (AD).

GARY'S PERSPECTIVE

Sue and PJ made a trip by bus to Albany with social workers
from the Alzheimer's Association. They visited the State Legisla-
ture, met with senators, and talked about Alzheimer's advocacy.
One issue Sue had to face was having the wrong words come out
when she tried to speak, but Sue knows exactly what she's trying
to say. Unfortunately, there is a disconnect somewhere—people
with Alzheimer's are misunderstood, but they do know what
they are trying to say.

Sue's short-term memory is becoming worse. It's difficult to
have a conversation because she loses thoughts. After a few tries,
Sue says, "Forget it." People need to be patient when talking with

someone with Alzheimer's. They often know what they want to say, just can't get the words out. People with Alzheimer's know more than they are given credit for. Sue has difficulty eating, cutting meat. Makes a mess around the plate, pushes things off. It's embarrassing for her. She doesn't always complete a task, for instance, closing a cabinet or drawer. Frustration for Sue is when she needs to say something and someone says, "Hold on." Most often, the thought is gone by the time that person is ready to listen.

Both PJ and Sue have trouble with numbers. For instance, when they went to lunch, the lunch check came, and they gave cash but had no idea how to figure tip, laughed quite a bit, and the waiter got a huge tip. Sue gets a haircut, uses a credit card, and asks store to add a 20% tip.

DYNAMICS OF OUR FAMILY

Our roles have changed. Sue used to coordinate all family functions. The disease is part of it, but so is technology. Sue can't text or read text. This makes the kids go to me all the time—this is upsetting to Sue. They do call her, but usually, day-to-day, it's texting.

Her inability to follow directions is a problem. Sue has always volunteered—can't do it anymore. She cannot follow directions well. Both Sue and PJ have the need to help others but cannot. They are trying to do so through Alzheimer's Association and taking part in speaking engagements about the disease.

Our daughter Kaitie was married in the spring and we traveled to South Carolina for the wedding. Sue was very anxious, but she didn't do anything to embarrass anyone. She ate very little for fear of making a mess. She learned from Kait's wedding what pitfalls to avoid at Ben's wedding in August.

In 2007, there were things that I now know were early warnings. Sue started bringing work schedules home to complete rather than finishing them at work. She knew what she wanted to do but just couldn't do it. She mentioned having difficulty with measuring and weighing patients and trouble filling in the charts.

This went on for a while, but it wasn't long before she decided it was time to leave work. Her fellow workers were very supportive of Sue during her decline. We followed their guidance to start the neurological ball rolling, and we thank them for all they did.

The next major difficulty for Sue was driving. At first, the sun bothered her eyes, then the rain, then headlights and darkness, and finally she started taking alternate routes to stay out of traffic. I ended up driving her to and from work and pretty much everywhere she went. She finally decided her eyes were not focusing well and stopped driving all together. Eye tests proved nothing, and we were told her eyes were fine.

Again, these items individually didn't seem to point in any direction. All the doctors had explained the symptoms as stress, menopause, exhaustion, and I think even the flu was blamed. Things got really bad in August of 2008. Sue went to her internist and was immediately referred for a neurological work up. I thought she may have had a stroke, as she was all right one day, and within a week, she could hardly function. Once the neurologist did a primary evaluation, we started the battery of tests. We went to tests every day, morning and afternoon, in hopes of finding something concrete. Unfortunately, the procedure currently is to rule things out, not diagnose.

DEMENTIA AS A FATAL DISEASE

Creutzfeldt-Jakob Disease (CJD) was mentioned as a possibility. I read all about it and couldn't believe what I was reading. CJD is a form of brain damage that leads to an extremely rapid decrease of mental function and movement. The disorder is fatal in a short time. I remember telling my best friend over a beer that I would take Alzheimer's in a minute if I could rule out CJD. Nobody knew about this possibility except me, and I went for almost three weeks thinking Sue had less than a year to live. I finally got the results of a spinal tap that ruled out CJD. I don't think I have ever told anyone about those three weeks until now. Remembering that time is very painful and I thank God for what we still have.

Creutzfeldt–Jakob disease (CJD) is a form of brain damage that leads to an extremely rapid decrease of mental function and movement. The disorder is fatal in a short time.... I went for almost three weeks thinking Sue had less than a year to live.

Sue continued to fail tests on a daily basis. On one test she couldn't even make sense of the example question. The administrator told me she had never had to deal with this problem before, so we went home and waited for the next test. In the meantime, Sue was started on Aricept, and things began improving almost as fast as they had gone downhill. Things still weren't normal, but the medications were helping and we adapted to our new lifestyle. Aricept seemed to be a miracle drug.

Our doctor started talking about Alzheimer's as a possible diagnosis but would not make a final diagnosis. We had pretty much gone as far as we could with him, and we went to Beth Israel Deaconess in Boston for a second opinion. That turned out to be our best decision so far. We went to a staff neurologist that specialized in Alzheimer's. After hours of testing and review of tests already taken, we finally got a diagnosis—posterior cortical atrophy (PCA). The doctor knew exactly what was wrong with her and now we did too. Unlike CJD, the symptoms of PCA develop more slowly than other kinds of dementia. It was really fun watching Dr. Press diagnose Sue. I had been at every appointment so far and I became familiar with the "tests" the specialists perform. I could see him run through his tests and start concentrating in a specific area, going away from that area, then circling back again. I could see him proving and disproving his theory. It was totally fascinating.

From the start, I have believed we were going to beat this thing, whatever it was. I now keep a totally upbeat attitude and don't think of the "downside." We have lived the last several years within our abilities. We still go out; we party with our family and with the friends that still call. We have a core group that is very supportive, but a lot of friends stopped calling. I imagine they were unsure of what to expect and are uncomfortable. That's hard on both of us, but especially Sue.

The truth is, Sue can do most things. She has trouble seeing and may be "legally" blind. She has trouble talking but always knows exactly what she wants to say. The words don't always cooperate. She needs help finding the food on her plate and maybe cutting a steak, but other than that she's a great date. She can't find the woman's room without help, but just point her in the right direction and she's fine. She doesn't do well with curbs and actually took a hard fall once when I looked away for a second, walking through a parking lot.

I help her dress every day that I'm home. If I'm not home she has clothes she can get on herself. I cook, clean, and do the laundry. We have a housekeeper that keeps things in order. Our three children are wonderful and totally supportive. When I'm out of town there are many people that help. The kids take turns having dinner with Sue and making sure everything is set before they leave. Kaitie is working on an exercise program for Sue to help keep her fit and the blood pumping.

All in all, life is good. I will take this illness over others and continue to believe a cure is almost here. People with Alzheimer's are people. Please don't forget that. Often they are more "with it" than you give them credit for. They just can't find the words when they need to. We have always finished each other's sentences; I'm sure due to our friendship since age 13. I can still finish Sue's sentences, which allows us to communicate even when Sue's words don't make sense.

The concern for Sue and PJ is that by talking about limitations, some will think they are complaining—not the case, just letting people know about the disease.

Sue's brother, Doug Taylor, offered his feelings about his sister's diagnosis, both as her brother and as a psychologist:

DOUG'S STORY

I've had such a range of reactions to Sue's illness since I became aware of her symptoms, and later, her diagnosis. I believe we first began talking about what was happening when she was having trouble at work. As she's described in this book, the symptoms were varied, but resulted in her no longer being able to do tasks that she had been competently doing for decades. Both of us have had our careers in health care. I could listen to her as a brother and as a psychologist, but I could only imagine the degree of frustration she must have been feeling as her ability to work slipped away. I was so hopeful at that stage that multiple sclerosis was the underlying problem. I knew there had been so much progress treating that disease.

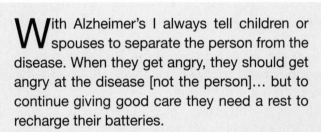

With Alzheimer's I always tell children or spouses to separate the person from the disease. When they get angry, they should get angry at the disease [not the person]... but to continue giving good care they need a rest to recharge their batteries.

DR. DANIEL Z. PRESS, NEUROLOGIST (WATSON, 2011)

As Sue continued to go through months of disappointing tests and appointments I began to seek out resources in Boston. I was able to locate Dr. Press; it was very helpful for me to be able to do something. Although dementia had been considered up to that point, it was still a shock when Alzheimer's was confirmed. I was glad Sue was past the anguish of living without an explanation, but so sad that she and her husband and children had to live with the illness. I became involved with the Alzheimer's Association and began to educate myself. The association funds a great deal of early research, which then leads to federally funded larger projects, so donations are very important. As a brother, gaining knowledge gives me something to focus upon, but doesn't relieve the sense of helplessness much.

For many of the months since Sue's diagnosis I did not see any noticeable changes in her when I traveled from Worcester to Syracuse. We would usually be together at her home, and our conversations were much like they always had been. I could see the roles changing in the family as Sue gradually did fewer tasks, but the visual and spatial problems did not stand out to me. More recently we went out to a bookstore together. Sue had difficulty negotiating the parking lot and was unsure how to operate the car door. That incident drove home the difficulties she was having. Lately I've noticed how she has begun to struggle with finding words. Sometimes she cannot organize what she wants to say. On other occasions we will have good talks about our extended family, but if facts are involved she may ask me to repeat them to Gary because she is not sure that she'll remember the details.

WHEN IT BECOMES TOO PERSONAL

Eight months ago I began to have some experiences that opened a window into Sue's world. I began to have cognitive trouble. For some time I had been joining my peers in their 50s and 60s as we complained about entering rooms and forgetting what we were after. Most of us were needing to use lists more and more. The changes that I began to notice were, however, different. At first I noticed that I could not organize my thoughts at times, though caffeine usually helped. Later, I began to have brief episodes in which I could not be sure where I was when I was driving—all the streets and the landscape seemed strange. I would have a vague hunch about which way to go, but without any confidence at all. Sometimes I just pulled over and called my wife. I knew that a small percentage of early onset Alzheimer's cases had a genetic basis and I became very afraid. Given that Dr. Press was Sue's neurologist, he saw me very quickly. This was followed by a battery of neuropsychological tests—strange to undergo, as I had administered many of them myself in the past. The outcome of this evaluation was the reassurance that I did not have dementia.

Dr. Press did suggest that I repeat a sleep study that I had undergone ten years prior. After that earlier study the neurologist I saw prescribed trazodone. I had continued to take that nightly for ten years. The new sleep specialist suggested that I taper off the medication. As I did, all of the worrisome symptoms cleared. I'm going into detail about this episode to make two points. First, until your mind stops working as it always has, I think it is impossible to taste the fear that early dementia causes. The second point is to stress how important it is to pay attention to cognitive symptoms and pursue a clear diagnosis. Many underlying causes can be addressed, and when a deteriorating neurological condition is the problem it can be important to start treatment as soon as possible.

When I've talked directly with Sue about her illness I have been so impressed by how she is coping with it. Her willingness to speak publicly to help others is such a gift and says so much about who she is as a person. Sue has a wonderful ability to make the best of things, a quality I grew up seeing in our mother. I know she gets frustrated and worried, but she seems to appreciate how critical it is to keep a positive outlook and take life as it comes. I'm reminded of a saying an elderly gentleman brought into a prostate cancer support group I once ran—"every day is a gift, that's why they call it the present." I go to Syracuse much more often than in years past and try to make the most of our visits together.

PJ's daughter, Tiffany, offers her thoughts on how the family has been coping with AD:

TIFFANY'S STORY

After Mom's diagnosis, there was a great sense of fear. What was to come? Mom and my stepfather moving to New York 1½ years ago was a relief! I was concerned about the depression that was hovering around my mom. Moving three blocks away from us was the key. I now was able to experience first-hand her mood of the day and figure out how I could help make things a bit easier. My goal since their relocation has been to keep her busy—outings for errands, helping out at our business, spending time with my daughters, and attending my girls' school events.

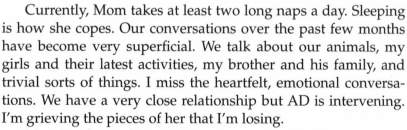

W e have a very close relationship, but AD is intervening. I'm grieving the pieces of her that I'm losing.

TIFFANY

Currently, Mom takes at least two long naps a day. Sleeping is how she copes. Our conversations over the past few months have become very superficial. We talk about our animals, my girls and their latest activities, my brother and his family, and trivial sorts of things. I miss the heartfelt, emotional conversations. We have a very close relationship but AD is intervening. I'm grieving the pieces of her that I'm losing.

Mom's relationship with Sue is wonderful. They compensate for each other's difficulties. My mom's short-term memory is severely impaired, whereas Sue remembers things short term. Sue has a tough time with words and my mom can fill in the blanks.

WHEN PATIENCE IS STRAINED

Patience is key. I find myself stopping to take a deep breath at times to get through a conversation we had only two minutes earlier. I watch Gary with Sue and have the utmost respect for the patience he has. He's so kind and has mastered the steps that help Sue complete a task.

Sue and PJ are very interested in finding a way to involve patients as well as caregivers in showing their feelings about Alzheimer's. In support groups, both patients and caregivers participate, but there are all levels of Alzheimer's, with some who have lost their ability to communicate verbally. Finding a way to reach them and giving those who are verbal an opportunity to speak their thoughts are priorities in a support group. The creative arts offer a base for communication with poetry, music, and art projects.

MAKING THE COMMITMENT

The Alzheimer's Association, a few meetings ago, had talked about who could be contacted and what kinds of places in which they could put pamphlets. The ideas they had were everything from general practitioners to banks. People in banks have to deal with people who have dementia. Mom knows the neurologist handles medications and the GP handles cholesterol, blood pressure, etc. She goes to Dr. Kittur, a local neurologist. She is very positive every time we're there, which is every three to six months, and she gives her little hints as far as staying positive, to not be so anxious. She gives her the mini mental exams. Her points awarded at the last two appointments have gone up, and Dr. Kittur is amazed.

Bob, PJ's husband, had trouble at first dealing with PJ's illness but eventually began to understand and support her.

BOB'S STORY

It is becoming quite common to see articles in the paper or magazines, not only about the Alzheimer's patient but also about their caregivers. Experiences with my wife, PJ, have been frustrating and difficult at times. However, I have generally been impressed by her being a model patient. It becomes trying when you are called on to answer the same question twenty times within three or four hours, but less difficult when your patient attempts to understand and continually apologizes for her confusion. It is then possible for the caregiver to be comforting rather than irritated, knowing how much she needs to be acknowledged. I often reassure her, "You don't have to apologize; you didn't ask for your disease."

The only time we had problems was right after she was first diagnosed. At the time, her cognitive abilities were being affected and it resulted in poor decisions on her part. I could not comprehend her actions and failed to relate them to her illness.

ACCEPTING CHANGE

However, I have to say at this point in her disease she is so thankful and appreciative of my support that I feel fully rewarded.

Dena Porter, Dave's daughter

DENA'S STORY

Dad seemed fine at the 50th anniversary celebration in July 2007. I didn't notice anything unusual that I remember during that time. I do remember Mom calling me from Mexico the following year in August to say Dad wasn't doing too well and was in the hospital in San Diego, and that he was confused about what was going on. She gave me the phone number for his room and I called him. That was the first time I noticed his confusion. He kept saying he just wanted to go home and why couldn't I just come and pick him up. It was hard to explain he wasn't in Pittsfield and would be home soon, just a plane ride away. It still wasn't real to me that Dad was having such problems.

When they did fly home, my brother Carl and I were at the airport to meet them. I couldn't wait to see my parents. They had been gone over a year and I needed to see them, to see Dad back home with all his family. Carl and I were waiting when someone came over to us to tell us that Dad was refusing to get off the plane. For him, the plane ride was too long with delays along the way, and it just made him more confused and anxious. They only let Carl go to the inner part of the airport because of security reasons. I just sat and cried, waiting to see what was happening to my father. I thought once he saw me, it would all be better—he would snap out of it.

When we were finally all together, my mother was still upset after the difficult plane ride, trying to calm him down, but when Carl and I appeared, he did seem to calm down a lot. The police and ambulance workers were there wanting us to take him to the hospital in Hartford (CT) but we wanted to take him to Pittsfield. We brought him home and admitted him to Berkshire Medical Center. I remember all he kept saying was he wanted to be home and didn't need to be in the hospital; he was just fine. It was hard for me but I knew I had to be strong. I went every day to see him and when he was discharged from the hospital, he had to go to a nursing home because their apartment wouldn't be ready for another month. I visited him at the nursing home every day, trying to keep him from forgetting, playing cards with him and walking the halls with him, sitting with him at dinner. He seemed to do pretty well when I was there. I did notice a difference, but he was still Dad, and no matter what he always would be. When he was doing better, we went out for rides. He seemed content, but got tired easily.

THE SOCIAL SIDE OF AD

Once Mom and Dad were in their apartment, we had a nice get-together at Christmas. On February 13, 2009, he and my twin grandchildren, Dante and Demetri, all celebrated their birthdays. Dad was 80 and the twins were 2 years old. We had a wonderful party at my house. I remember Dad was playing with one of the boys, tapping a balloon back and forth. He loved being with the family. After that, however, he seemed to get more tired physically and mentally. It was very hard on Mom over the next three weeks until he passed. I knew when the phone rang that Mom was not able to calm him down, and I would go over to try and help. The last night was so hard. The firemen came to help out. He wouldn't take his medicine and the oxygen line wouldn't stay under his nose. My mother and I tried to get him into bed, but we couldn't move him. The firemen made him comfortable. At some time during the night, however, he made his journey to heaven. He will be remembered always, with love.

Dave's son Carl relates his story.

CARL'S STORY

My relationship with my father has always been a simple one. We loved and respected each other; that's it, and although I have given him reasons to change that position, he has never given me anything but love, with just the right amount of discipline.

Time spent with him was predictable, in that I understood where he was coming from; it made sense, we understood each other. I never saw fear or confusion in my father's face. He always knew what needed to be done and how to do it and would take on any problem or project without worry of failure. This is the side he must have wanted us to see. My father's intelligence,

71

great sense of humor, and friendly smile were his three biggest attributes and the ones least likely to be affected, so I thought.

RECOGNIZING THE DISEASE

Alzheimer's introduced fear, worry, and confusion to a life that had little experience with those things, and he was in no position to learn a new way. His passing was on his terms, and thanks to proper medication and support from the family, he left us with all the important memories intact.

Dave's older son John speaks.

JOHN'S STORY

Dad was always a quiet guy. He could be the life of a party, but usually he was simply a quiet presence. There were no deep, philosophical discussions. No ponderings of life's mysteries. He was always so happy to see me, I never doubted for one minute that he loved me. Yet I felt that I never really knew the guy inside David Allen. But Mom was so deep, philosophical, and multidimensional that I just accepted the balanced package.

Jill and I made a real connection with Dad at the 50th wedding anniversary party. Dad seemed to fully appreciate the similarities between the American House—our Bed and Breakfast at the time—and my grandmother's house, where he had grown up, both in physical similarities as well as a common energy, or aura. Particularly during the anniversary party, with the house full of family bustling from room to room, love and a sense of family abounded and overflowed the house! I remember Dad, while sitting in a chair, just taking in the similarities, said, with a smile, "I feel like I'm in Gaga's house!" Now, Mom, who was beginning to suspect changes in Dad, said, in a worried tone, "Now David, you know that you are not in your mother's house, this is John's house." And of course Dad, in a very irritated tone, responded, "I know that!" Because I clearly saw that Mom had totally misread that precious moment, I, from that point forward, became suspect of the accuracy of her diagnosis of Dad.

GROWING PHYSICAL PROBLEMS

I had very limited exposure to Dad, as they were in Mexico off and on for many years. And after their return, Dad always knew exactly who I was, though he did have a tendency to confuse my wife Jill with my ex-wife, Deirdre. I clearly saw his physical demise, and because of that, I now commit to regular stretching and exercise so as not to walk in those footprints. I guess the bottom line for me is that his disease was not apparent to me; only the physical deterioration stood out.

Stories from Later Stages in the Disease Process

*S*ue and PJ's family members continue to document their struggles and observations about the way in which Alzheimer's disease (AD) has impacted them and their loved ones. For Sue and PJ, 2011 was a year of change, not so much with their illness but with a drastic change in what was familiar. They depended on each other, but now they are no longer able to meet, although they stay in touch by phone. Sue became a grandmother and lost both her mother and father. PJ and Bob moved to Canada in summer and Florida in winter, and PJ was physically separated from Sue as well as from her daughter, Tiffany. In addition, PJ's son, Char, lost his life in a snowmobile accident, and the family has been going through a difficult time with this loss, especially PJ.

GARY

It's been almost five years since this all began. Doctors at the time told us that five years was about the time we would have before Sue was under total care at a nursing home or somewhere.

The time has flown by and Sue needs help with pretty much everything she does. I put the toothpaste on but she brushes. I help her wash and dress. Someone gets all her meals. She can't read, write, or spell. She can't dial the phone or change the TV channel. She has trouble opening and closing the sliding door to let the dogs out. I worry that if she's alone she may not be able to get out of the house if she needed to. With all of her limitations, she is in a happy place. Nothing seems to bother her too much; she's rarely sad. When she is sad it's usually about someone else's problems.

She loves to hold our granddaughter Abbie and play with her too. She can joke with me, watches TV, and tries to read. She keeps asking for new magazines and books because she's "read all the old ones." I keep buying them but they just sit. I'm sure I don't notice her lack of ability as much as others who don't see her as often. I know eating out has gotten tougher. Last week she wanted a glass of wine with dinner. I asked the waitress to put it in a glass with no stem. She tends to not be able to set it down without spilling. I usually guide it to the table but it's easier to get rid of the stem. Coffee cups are sometimes too heavy and nothing can be filled to the top or it will spill. I cut up her food and tell her where things are on the plate. We have a nice time but it's a challenge now. Often parts of dinner end up on the floor or on her. It's becoming easier to eat home. I'm a pretty good cook. I've gotten better recently and Sue's always ready to try my latest recipe. We have a few regular spots we go where the waitresses know us and take very good care of us.

Sue can't find the car door very well anymore. I open it and she has trouble deciding which leg to put in first. Once she's in I hook her seatbelt and we're off to somewhere.

I noticed several years ago that Sue does things opposite of what you ask or expect. If I tell her to sit she stands, left is right, etc. I originally thought it was strange because we all make an occasional mistake, but she does the opposite almost 99% of the time. It's a part of the disease that I wasn't expecting and it makes asking her to do something difficult. She has also starting to put things away in different places. We're still looking for her hair brush, lipsticks, and several other things. We can laugh about it, but it's frustrating to me.

CAREGIVER STRESS

I have become excessively "efficient" with my time. My children say I have OCD. Time is so valuable when trying to work, run a house, and care for my family and Sue. I have no time for mistakes or anything slow. Seeing me run around the grocery store must be quite a sight. I carefully plan my list so I don't backtrack, and then selecting the correct checkout line and getting upset with myself if I have made the wrong choice. In the house I plan things out so that I don't take extra steps. Things will pile up near the stairs so I can carry as much as possible with each trip. That way I don't make additional trips. I entertain myself by planning out my day and trying to be as efficient as I can, but truthfully sometimes I take it too far.

We had one of our bathrooms remodeled in the house. It's on the main floor and next to our new bedroom. We looked at the patio home idea to get everything on one floor, but I really couldn't give up my backyard, especially with grandchildren here and on the way. We figured we would remodel the house so that everything that Sue needed was on one floor. We took out the tub and put in a walk-in shower. We added handrails and a seat. So far it's working out well, but Sue still can't handle the water temperature and I'm afraid she'll burn herself so I facilitate the shower. We moved from our upstairs bedroom to the room next to the bathroom. We got some new furniture, curtains, and a fresh coat of paint. It's a "new to us" room.

We'll continue to remodel throughout the year until our old home is freshened up and suits our needs.

Our friends are very interested in how Sue's doing. I have no problems talking to anyone about Sue until they ask about me. "So, how are you holding up?" shuts me down every time. I don't want to talk about me so please don't ask. I can deal with each day; I have help so I can travel for work and also work in my office in the house. I get out to play golf once a week in a league that I've been in for 14 plus years. That is my most enjoyable day of the week.

I've been told by several friends and family that I should get therapy, talk to someone, or "get help." Truth is, if I had time for therapy I'd use it to play more golf. It's just more time consumption that I don't have.

I talk to friends when I want to. Old friends seem to work best for me. A lot of them have known Sue and me since 7th grade or even longer—others not so long. I talk when I feel like it, not when someone else wants me to. Sometimes I email with a friend in California. I find that email allows me to say things I wouldn't say face to face. I used to be quite an emotional person, not as bad now but I still cry at "Lion King." I hammer away at the keyboard and I get out some of my feelings and emotions. It feels good, it helps a lot, and my friend always sends back a positive, character-building response. That and the occasional beers with Joe is all I need for now.

I'll be fine.

I wish our children would seek help. I ask them to talk about their feelings or concerns with me. Nobody wants to talk much, although this whole thing has to be hard on them all. I hope they are at least talking to each other, but I don't know. They all seem to be most worried about me. I try to tell them that I'm fine, but they don't seem to accept that.

Sue and I have been married 35 years this year. We have had more time together than most married couples our age. In addition, we were best friends for 8 years before that. I'm used to caring for her and I always will. Of our friends, we were always the ones that did things first. First to get married, first to buy a house, first to have a baby, the list goes on. We are not the first to deal with personal illness, but we're in the top few.

The bathroom still is the largest challenge for us when we go anywhere. Sue can no longer manage the door or the stall by herself. She has gotten stuck in restrooms at places and I have had to get someone to help. She takes care of personal business but can't manage the doors. Lately we can only go places that are between bathroom visits. That makes travel more difficult, and although most state rest stops have a "family restroom," many still do not. A few other places have family restrooms, but I imagine with the increase in Alzheimer's and other dementias, this will become easier as time goes on. We are now flying to our vacations. That's not unusual for most families, but I hate to fly and I love to drive. I feel I'm on vacation as soon as I start out on the trip when I drive. Not so much when I fly.

We are trying to plan a 35th wedding anniversary trip this year. Our first choice would be to rent a house on the ocean somewhere and have all the children come to somewhere warm and have family time for a week. It's not so easy anymore with everyone's schedule, but we're hoping we can pull it off. Our next choice is to go somewhere with friends or at least go somewhere by ourselves. We'll see what happens.

Sue's speech has gotten much worse recently. It's hard to tell what she wants or what she's trying to say. I ask questions and sometimes I can get it, other times she gets frustrated and says "never mind." It really bothers me when she gives up. I know it's frustrating to her and I still say she knows exactly what she wants to say; the words just don't come out right. When we see people we know, I tell her who they are before they get close to us. She wouldn't know them if I didn't tell her. Several months ago, we talked with a few friends for 10 minutes, and when they left she asked, "Who were those people?" Once I told her who they were, she knew them and wished she had known earlier so she could have been more into the conversation. Sue is aware of those issues and therefore doesn't want to go out in public where she might not recognize someone. This is just another part of the disease that isolates you and is not written about in medical books.

Every night when I'm falling to sleep I think of winning the lottery. It's fun for me to escape reality and think "what if?" Because it's an escape I don't think of winning a million, I think big. $300,000,000 is a personal favorite, sometimes even more. The number one thing I would do is buy a Bentley convertible. Sorry, that's just me. Number two would be to make sure our children were financially set for the rest of their lives. The number three thing would be to help find a cure for this disease. I read of medical advances but they never seem to mature. I have to believe there is a cure to be found within our lifetime. We just need to uncover it.

That's all I have.

SUE'S BROTHER DOUG

It is the beginning of a new year. The seven months since I first wrote a contribution to this evolving book have been long and trying for our family.

One of the very good things about this time period is that Sue has remained mostly as she was in May. We, along with our spouses, have coped together with our father's decline as he showed increasing signs of Alzheimer's and a deteriorating neurological disease that was a variation of ALS. He died one month ago. While Sue continued through the year to slowly develop more trouble articulating her thoughts, I was able to trust that she clearly understood all the issues we faced. We were able to make decisions together during my father's month-long hospitalization, including which treatments to refuse, and ultimately when to shift to comfort care and hospice. As I look back upon my experience, I realize that I did not perceive Sue as an Alzheimer's patient, but more as my sister who now had visual and speech disabilities. In our many trips to the hospital, we developed a routine for her to successfully get in and out of my car. Initially, the decisions about how she should position herself and which limb to move next seemed very taxing. With practice this was not a problem. I did find it hard to see her frustration when she had trouble remembering nursing terms that she'd used for years. While we both wished that we could have done more for my father, I think our helplessness was especially hard for her.

I was always invited to Sue and Gary's for dinner during the many trips to Syracuse. Sharing a meal gave us all the opportunity to relax some, reminisce, plan, and talk about the other parts of our lives. It's been especially enjoyable for me to watch Sue's pleasure in becoming a grandmother. As our children become the adults we so recently became ourselves, it's good to be able to enjoy family life together.

PJ'S 15-YEAR OLD GRANDDAUGHTER JENNA

PJ is my grandmother. She has been my grandmother, who I call Meme, for as long as I remember. She has always been there for me no matter what. Although she doesn't have the best memory anymore, she still has the biggest heart. She has changed a little over the years, but not how you would think a person would change. She did not change her hair or her clothes. It isn't that kind of change; it is more of an internal change. It wasn't her personality either. She changed because of Alzheimer's.

It isn't the kind of disease that you can just look at and see she has it. She is still the same person and has the same fun-loving and kind-hearted personality, just with less of a memory. A passerby on the street or a person she goes up to and talks to, because she loves meeting new people, might just think, "She is such a nice woman." You can only notice when you are trying to talk to her, and even then it isn't that noticeable. But to those who have known her for a long time like me and my family it is noticeable, but we push through and support her because we know how hard it is for us, and it must be even harder for her. Sometimes we get frustrated, but we are human; we just keep remembering that this is our Meme and that she is the same Meme we have always had and have always loved.

PJ'S DAUGHTER TIFFANY

My family and I went to visit my brother Char in December for a week in Rochester, Minnesota, as they had relocated there in October from Phoenix, Arizona. My brother was able to be a stay-at-home dad temporarily while they got settled. While in Minnesota visiting, Char and I had some awesome bonding time and talked a lot about Mom and our thoughts of the future. He agreed to write a piece for this book when he "had a chance... soon." He never got the chance. Char was killed in a snowmobile accident on January 28th, 2012. Our lives will never be the same.

One my best conversations with my brother was what we had learned from our mom and how it has gotten us through life. At very early ages we picked up on Mom's love for reading. We weren't big television watchers and preferred to read, especially before going to bed. We love non-fiction and fiction. Our mom would frequently send books to us with a sweet passage or some words of wisdom. Until six months ago, she was still sending books to us and to our children.

Our mom is a bit of a "reactor," and safety was always and still is a big concern of hers for us and those around her. We were always told by her to "scan our environment" and know always what was happening around us. Another favorite was, "Use your head; don't do anything stupid or reckless." It's a wonder we were ever allowed to do anything! It was always meant to keep us safe.

My mom moved to Canada in April 2011 with my stepfather, Bob. The idea was to take advantage of free health care and free long-term care. They rented an apartment in Prescott, Ontario, on the St. Lawrence River. Mom loved the view but felt very isolated, as the only people around were Bob's son and daughter-in-law. Her cats were the one constant and source of comfort. I frequently tried to get her to visit us in Syracuse, which she thought was great. However, this past year, when the day to visit approached, she was unsure and thought she would just come for a day. This went on all summer. We talked daily and had grand ideas for visits, but she felt better being in Canada. I believe she was overwhelmed about getting things ready for the visit.

Bob decided in September that they would spend time at Bob's daughter and son-in-law's condo in Davie, Florida. The change again impacted my mom. The stress of the drive was tremendous and getting to a new place was confusing. After she was there for a few days, our conversations moved to her repeatedly asking me when they would return to Canada. Mom focused on the fact that she missed her cats in Canada terribly and that the neighbors in the condo community were nowhere to be seen. She would spend most of her time out on the lanai area looking at the surrounding condos. She constantly remarked that there was nobody around, no lights on. They stayed until the week before Christmas and returned to Canada.

On their way back, Mom stayed the night with us and Bob returned to Canada. She was anxious and unsure of "the plan" to get back home. It was great to have her with us and we enjoyed our short time together. The bedtime routine went well. At about 4:00 a.m. I heard her wandering—took me right back to being a kid and finding her sleepwalking! She was awake, had gone to the bathroom, and forgot which room she was in. Back to bed.

The next day was tough. Mom kept asking what the plan was and when she needed to be ready. I told her to shower and get dressed and off we'd go to meet Bob. She looked at me and said, "What do I do first?" We went through the routine step by step. She can still shower and wash herself, but getting the towel and turning on the shower was difficult and frustrating for her. Clothes are also a big deal. She is conscientious about trying not to wear the same outfit and the picking out process is taxing.

She returned to Canada with Bob and lo and behold a new residence! Bob's son owned a rental house in Prescott and Mom and Bob decided to rent it, as they didn't like being in an apartment situation. Another change and more stress. The new place is not on the river but allows them some more privacy. Mom actually said she felt good there, and Bob's son and daughter-in-law had completely moved their things from the apartment to the house while they were in Florida. Mom seemed happy but began dreading the trip back to Florida.

Mom and Bob returned to Florida in 2012. Again, Mom was not excited and felt horrible about leaving her cats. Bob's daughter's family has cat allergies, so having them in Florida was not an option. Bob's daughter, Lee, spends most of her time in California at her other home, which allowed Mom and Bob the condo to themselves except when Lee came for short stays.

This time, while in Florida, it took my mom only two days to ask when she would return to Canada. We joked about that. I'd ask her if she wanted the truth or should I make up a time; she'd say, make it up! She actually liked the idea of the little house in Canada and had big plans for gardens she'd plant in the spring. Again, her focus was on the lack of people in the condo community. She'd frequently ask why she complained, since most people would give their right arm to be in such a place with warmth and sunshine.

I know what my pain is—having lost my brother. I can't imagine what it's like for my mom and my dad. Our lives are forever changed. I truly thought this tragedy would make my mom snap. I can't describe the sounds she made when I called to tell her. It was a guttural, sobbing, heart-wrenching moan that I hope to never hear again. Her world had crashed and nobody could explain why.

She understood and still understands that it happened and the grief comes in waves at bizarre times. For the first few days after the accident, she would wake up at night and go to the lanai and cry. Bob would go out and try to get her back to bed. She'd ask him why she was so sad and upset and needed to know who she was grieving for. Mom had to relive the horror as he reminded her it was Char she was grieving for.

Weeks after Char's death, Mom and I still talk at least every other day as we always have. She has good days and bad days. While we were in Minnesota two weeks ago, Bob and I discussed my mom and I asked him to support me in encouraging Mom to visit more often for a day or two at a time. She is in definite agreement as is he. Bob says that it's getting more difficult to take care of her. I think the repeating of things and questions are grueling for him and I'm happy to share the responsibility with him. Since they moved to Canada last year, I continue to send all of her prescriptions, prepare them, and mark them by the week. They both are unable to sort and organize them and at times I know Bob forgets to remind her to take them. I know that he tries his best.

They plan on returning here the first week of March and we are all really looking forward to it. We all miss Meme.

Our conversations now are about my brother and the great memories we have. She worries constantly about Brenda and her two youngest grandchildren. When I ask my mom how she feels, she says that she is coasting, that she should be gone, not her son.

We talk about how unfair life is and how we don't understand why this tragedy has happened. I worry about depression setting in and am trying to keep a close eye on her mood. Mom continues her negative self-talk. It's difficult to change because it is part of her personality. She is very hard on herself and frequently refers to herself as a nit-wit. We correct her constantly and redirect the conversation. I know my brother had a tough time during conversations with my mom because the negative talk is so very negative. It's hard to change the pattern and turn it into a positive.

When I've asked my mom about her Alzheimer's diagnosis and what she wants people to know, she is very excited about this book as it shares her story. She says that there's a little voice in her head that constantly corrects her and tells her to "straighten up, get it right." The pressure she puts on herself must be exhausting for her. While in Minnesota the first week of February for my brother's services, people were amazed. "Your mom looks great." "She's doing so well." Patronizing, as Mom would say. She'd wonder what she's supposed to "look like," and would say that if she knew what others had said. The picture most people have in their minds of someone with Alzheimer's is a non-communicating, or rambling individual who was maybe acting inappropriately. Not true at this point!

We don't know what the future will bring. I know that I can never let my mom go into a "home" when Bob can no longer take care of her, especially three hours away, in another country. She will come live with us and I will care for her as long as I'm able and my family is willing. My family; husband, Eric; daughters, and friends are a terrific support. Char was my sounding board and was a fantastic listener when I was frustrated or needed to vent about the day or about conversations with our mom. I can't even express how much I miss him....

8

Getting Help in the Home or in a Facility

MAINTAINING QUALITY OF LIFE

Alan Dienstag's article (2010) on ways to improve the quality of life for Alzheimer's patients in a support group or nursing home notes that it is one thing to have Alzheimer's at an older age, when health problems take precedence and Alzheimer-type symptoms are apt to be blamed on physical deterioration—these patients are either never told they have Alzheimer's or are unable to communicate whether they understand the implications of having the disease—it's quite something else when those in the early stages do know what the diagnosis means and have yet to lose their ability to communicate.

One of the most important aspects of treating Alzheimer's is finding a way to keep the person involved and interested. Dienstag presented several challenges for those who have the disease and those caring for them:

1. Therapy for Alzheimer patients and their families: quilting, painting, ceramics, poetry, and music. It offers a way to help express feelings and improve quality of life.

2. The challenge is to construct a life in the shadow of an advancing disease.

3. It is important to be positive rather than negative about the disease. Don't be defined by what you *can't* do; consider what you *can* do.

4. Writing, as noted in Dienstag's article, can be utilized as therapy, asking members of a support group to express their feelings and appointing someone to either record or take notes on what is being said. According to Don DeLillo, an author whose mother-in-law has Alzheimer's disease (AD), "Writing is a form of memory."

5. It is important for members of a support group and staff in a nursing home to be aware of and understand the diagnosis so that they can deal with it.

6. Support groups for caregivers are very necessary, but support groups specifically for those with early stage AD are largely absent.

For those wanting to consider a group for early stage AD, the following areas can offer suggestions:

Senior Centers—While Alz.org offers chapters throughout the country and abroad, senior centers offer local information and assistance for those dealing with dementia, mostly age-related type (activities and adult day care programs), as well as meeting with caregivers. At present, the focus is on caregivers rather than those in the early stage of the disease, and there is a need to communicate with others in the same situation.

Elder Services—This state-sponsored organization is available for those over 60 and guides them through various programs, including

(continued)

housing, medical care, assessment, home care, nursing homes, and Alzheimer's care, and also serves individuals under 60 in certain programs. When my husband and I first moved back to Pittsfield, Bea Cowlin, an advocate for seniors at Elder Services in Pittsfield, helped us with health care and housing, and introduced me to an overwhelming number of books about Alzheimer's.

LOSS OF INCOME

Perhaps the area that touches almost everyone is money. Even in an economy that has caused massive unemployment, people tend to take their income for granted. As long as they are willing to work or be available for work, they are convinced the money will come in. They might have an unexpected job loss, but it's expected to be temporary until they find another job.

But what happens if a person loses the ability to do his or her job or any other job and has no idea why? What if it is necessary to stop working with no chance of returning to the job that person has been trained to do, at a time when most people start looking forward to retirement? For some reason, most of the stories that show up written by those with the disease or about Alzheimer's have to do with those at the higher end of the education ladder, and often with those in the medical or teaching fields. Losing part of the population to AD is a tragedy because those who have it can no longer fulfill their potential.

This is the case with Sue and P.J. and they have shared with me not only how they have coped with the disease, but especially from income loss.

Sue—I had to quit work at 52. I worked for 18 years part time around our children. As Lizzie, our youngest, got older, I worked more and more so that I was up to 30 to 35 hours per week for the last few years. The financial impact of Alzheimer's on our family was the total loss of my salary. Our savings suffered first and then our ability to retire. My early constant medical testing was both time consuming and expensive. We were feeding our 401K as much as possible in order to someday retire. Now, the ability to retire is a long way off at best, and the need for medical insurance makes it a necessity for Gary to keep working past retirement age. Social security disability insurance is available to those diagnosed with Alzheimer's, but getting the diagnosis is difficult and takes a long time. I could never do the paperwork myself and, fortunately, Gary was able to do it and get me approved. Some have to use lawyers and often the first request is denied. The overall time frame, start to finish, was over a year. I get about 25% of what I was making, and although it helps, it could not support me if anything happened to Gary, especially since I already need a caregiver.

PJ—My husband is a golfer. Once he retired, he just immersed himself in golf. I supported him in that, but I hate golf. Bob, however, takes care of all finances—he's an accountant—and even though I had to stop working, I don't think we had or yet have any financial problems. I had already retired from Cornell University and of course Bob was retired. I immersed myself in reading and socializing, and when I began having cognitive problems, I tried to represent myself on paper regarding what I was going through. I spent a lot of time staring into space. My problem was not money. It was depression. And sometimes it becomes overwhelming. We're looking for speaking engagements and working on this book to educate the public about this debilitating disease.

Dave—For close to ten years, Dave gradually became more and more confused, with increased medical problems that required trips to the states from Mexico, where we spent part of every year. The last year we spent on the Baja in Mexico, Dave had to be transported twice by ambulance to the border, and from there to El Centro, California, and finally by helicopter to Scripps Green Hospital in San Diego. The expense of this was extreme because insurance didn't cover all of it. We also had to pay medical bills in Mexico because we weren't covered by insurance there. By the time we accepted the fact that we had to return to Massachusetts, our only recourse financially was to declare bankruptcy. We started proceedings the beginning of 2008 and finalized them in the fall of 2008—I had to fly back to El Centro to attend court and my son, Carl, accompanied me. Even so, our only income was Social Security and Dave needed several prescriptions filled every month. Also, it was necessary for me to set up a payment plan for Dave's physician for amounts not covered by insurance. I am finally on a working budget with very little extra every month. I do work for the local paper as an obituary clerk a couple of days a week, and that helps.

WHAT DOES THE FUTURE HOLD?

One problem for women that complicates a diagnosis of early onset AD is the onset of menopause, often blamed for symptoms. Also, the family is apt to be in denial, which creates a lack of support. One of the earliest symptoms of dementia is loss of cooking abilities, which can create dangerous situations when a stove is left on under a pan or a mix of cleaning chemicals causes a noxious gas. Time becomes a major focus for those with AD. Everything takes longer and there is such a concern that appointments will be forgotten that they are ready hours before the appointment. Just getting dressed in the morning can take a very long time. As we move further into the 21st century, it becomes more evident that the costs related to Alzheimer's and other dementias will increase greatly, especially for families trying to care for loved ones at home.

This is why humor helps in dealing with a disease that is far from humorous. Being connected to another person who has early onset offers the opportunity to share the common difficulties faced with both humor and acceptance. One such difficulty is the frustration of not being able to do things previously taken for granted. Another is the concern about time and forgetting an appointment or a meeting. Accepting the limitations brought about by AD is difficult but imperative. It is necessary to avoid stressful situations. When in the company of those whose thinking is not impaired, it becomes obvious they don't understand what is happening to you. They become impatient and you become frustrated.

AD is a disease that changes your daily routine. A diagnosis creates the feeling that no one, not even family members, really understands what is happening to you. This is a case where being able to communicate with another person who has been diagnosed leads to acceptance as well as the ability to share problems in a humorous way. When three people are seated at a table and one of them has early stage AD, the other two hesitate to take a humorous viewpoint and have trouble accepting such a diagnosis from someone who seems so normal. But if three people are seated at a table and they all have early stage, humor abounds. They understand each other. The more we, the public, understand about this disease, the better we will be able to deal with it. Sue and PJ are able to communicate well with each other, and finding humor in everyday life by sharing their various foibles keeps them active and accepting.

The Alzheimer's Association has the right idea about trying to educate the public about the disease; however, not everyone spends time keeping up by joining one of their sites. Unless a person has been diagnosed with the disease or is caregiver of a person with the disease, it is unlikely that person will even enter Alz.org or local Alzheimer's sites. On the other hand, the number of people with Alzheimer's is increasing at such a rate that finding a way to make the general public want to know more is imperative. In a country where Levi Johnson (unwed father of Sarah Palin's grandson) became a household name, at least long enough to garner 3,000,000 hits on his site in one day, with only 357,000 the same day for early onset Alzheimer's, what does it take to make millions of people click on Alz.org? We all know someone who has Alzheimer's but we don't know much about the disease itself. To create a media flurry, unfortunately, there has to be conflict and controversy. This book, along with the annotated bibliography below, gives a view of AD that educates the public about aspects of this disease not previously known by most people. One book does not have all the answers, but several books in the following bibliography offer an overview that touches almost everyone facing this disease as either patient or caregiver or family and friends.

ANNOTATED BIBLIOGRAPHY

Castleman, Michael, Gallagher-Thompson, Dolores, and Naythons, Matthew. *There's Still a Person In There: The Complete Guide to Treating and Coping with Alzheimer's*. New York: G.P. Putnam's Sons, 2000. This is a collection of personal and professional vignettes describing the effects of Alzheimer's on the population. The practical advice in this book continues to be relevant more than ten years after publication. It covers the way the disease affects different people and how families cope with its progression. Here is a book that moves beyond the diagnosis and offers ways to accept what might be ahead by living life a day at a time.

Cooney, Eleanor. *Death in Slow Motion: My Mother's Descent Into Alzheimer's*. New York: HarperCollins, 2003. Cooney's method of coping with her mother's Alzheimer's was for her to turn to drink and drugs, which, of course, made the disease more hers than her mother's. Her mother had established a reality that worked for her but created great difficulty for her daughter. This is a story of how a caregiver might deal with Alzheimer's in a loved one when the caregiver has trouble creating a life style that accepts the disease. Much of the text in the book deals with Cooney's efforts to reason with her mother's bizarre comments instead of just accepting them. Cooney says, "I tried to put myself in her mind, but I couldn't. She was on a different planet."

DeBaggio, Thomas. *Losing My Mind: An Intimate Look at Life with Alzheimer's*. New York: Simon & Schuster, 2002. This is one of the few books written from the viewpoint of a person with Alzheimer's. It is difficult for the public to accept the fact that those with the disease can communicate so well, but DeBaggio proves it to be the case. He alternates from his herb growing experiences to his past personal memories and his current life with Alzheimer's. DeBaggio has an excellent command of language and the book is musical and educational. He has recently followed this book with *When It Gets Dark: An Enlightened Reflection on Life with Alzheimer's* (2007).

Genova, Lisa. *Still Alice*. New York: Simon and Schuster, January, 2009. Here are two years in the life of a woman with early onset Alzheimer's. Genova makes the main character in this novel, Alice Howland, as real as any person actually dealing with this disease, but Alice is a fictional character. It's true that Genova does not have Alzheimer's in any form, but her insight into the disease through her creation of Alice is truly remarkable and makes this story both first-person and subjective. She begins the story with Alice leading a normal life, teaching and lecturing in college, and gradually shows how early onset Alzheimer's is manifesting itself. It reads like first person but is actually told by the narrator, Genova. This is a highly recommended book for anyone who is trying to understand the disease.

King, James. *Bill Warrington's Last Chance*. New York, Viking, 2010. This novel introduces a man in his seventies who begins to show signs of dementia and then moves into the story of a dysfunctional family, consisting of Bill Warrington's two sons, daughter, and granddaughter. It is the granddaughter, April, who connects to and cares about her grandfather, while the rest of the family is focused on themselves. She and Bill impulsively leave on a trip cross country, April to realize her dream of going to San Francisco and Grandpa to force his three children to finally get together. For April, the trip is a coming of age and for her grandfather a gradual journey further into dementia. Occasionally, at the beginning of the story, Bill's point of view lacks authenticity, but as the story progresses, April and Bill's interaction is valid, and the conclusion is satisfying.

Koenig-Coste, Joanne. *Learning to Speak Alzheimer's. (Mariner Books)* New York: Houghton Mifflin, 2004. Much of this book is clinical, with specific information on symptoms, diagnosis, and suggestions on how to interact with those who have Alzheimer's. For instance, "If I can reach him on an emotional level … instead of on a verbal or cognitive one, maybe life will be less threatening for him."

Mobley, Tracy. *Young Hope: The Broken Road*. Denver, Colo.: Outskirts Press, Inc., 2007. The author chose to write about her own experiences with early onset Alzheimer's disease, but grammatical errors made the book difficult to read at times. A copy editor would have been most helpful. However, her story is extremely important at a time when too little is known about early onset AD. Tracy was diagnosed in 2002 at the age of 38. She began writing this book, which was published four years later when she was 42, too young to collect disability through Social Security. Even now, when being eligible requires the applicant to be at least 50, Tracy is still in her 40s. Tracy notes that there has to be "something to bring more focus, not only on the disease but to the faces" to show that this is not an "old" person's disease.

Montgomery, Michelle. *Alzheimer Diary: A Wife's Journey.* Newton, MA: WorldMaker Media, 2010. The author is the caregiver here. Her husband has Alzheimer's. Unfortunately, her first paragraph speaks of her husband going out and being gone so long, she begins to worry. But she doesn't close out the experience. How long was he gone? Was he all right? There are perhaps more questions than answers in this diary. How old is her husband? She has grown children, sometimes cares for her 4-year-old granddaughter, but no one seems to be relieving her. Why not? This is a generalized look at Alzheimer's disease as it affects the caregiver.

Peterson, Betsy. *Voices of Alzheimer's: Courage, Humor, Hope and Love in the Face of Dementia.* Cambridge, MA: Da Capo Press, 2004. This book is a series of short quotations collected by the author from patients and caregivers regarding everything from being diagnosed with Alzheimer's to facing changes in routine, loneliness, support groups, money worries, and finally the end stages of the disease. It's similar to a mini-encyclopedia and is useful for anyone starting to deal with dementia and hearing about the progression from those who are at different stages.

Smith, Amber. "A family faces Alzheimer's disease: Central New York mother and daughter become patient and caregiver." *The Post Standard.* 9/21/2010. The article was written by Smith during an interview with PJ Kimmerly, one of the authors of this book, and her daughter, Tiffany, as a means of educating the public about early onset Alzheimer's disease. http://blog.syracuse.com/cny/2010/09/a_family_faces_alzheimers_disease

Taylor, Richard. *Alzheimer's from the Inside Out.* Baltimore: Health Professions Press, 2007. Taylor's background and creative talent makes him eminently successful in telling the story of his illness.

It also shows the public that to have early onset Alzheimer's disease does not take away the ability to communicate, at least throughout the first five years after diagnosis. Taylor's wry sense of humor is immediately evident. It's easy to forget why Taylor is writing these essays (to educate the public) and just enjoy his writing style. This is an honest look at a devastating disease.

Young, Ellen P. *Between Two Worlds: Special Moments of Alzheimer's and Dementia.* Amherst, NY: Prometheus Books, 1999. Here is a collection of interviews and vignettes collected by Young as she shares her experiences with family and clients and shows that there is a life after a diagnosis of Alzheimer's disease. What is missing, however, are the voices of Alzheimer's, the personal viewpoint of people who have the disease. One chapter, "Tommy Thompson," is written by the author about her interview with Tommy, who has early onset, but as with the rest of the book, the viewpoint is Ellen's.

DIFFERENT ASPECTS OF WRITING ABOUT AD

For anyone who has Alzheimer's and tries to organize and write about it without professional assistance as it progresses, the energy needed to do this is overwhelming and very time-consuming. It can be done, as shown by Mobley, who made a point of doing it all herself, and DeBaggio, who created his own way of organizing his thoughts, and by Genova, by creating a character with early onset AD based on her many years of inter-action with the disease. Taylor wrote about his experience in a series of essays written over a five-year period. When my husband's niece, Sue, expressed an interest in writing a book about AD with her friend, PJ, I collected their thoughts and experiences and discovered how important their friendship is in dealing with such a lonely disease. Their input led me to read several books about the personal aspects of Alzheimer's and access several sites about Alzheimer's online, which helped me organize material for this book, along with their amazing input.

96

Just about any book I have read from the caregiver's viewpoint has been more about the caregiver than the patient. This goes for *Jan's Story* (2010) by Barry Peterson, which was definitely more about him and his needs. With the online video, he made a great effort to justify having a girlfriend while his wife was alive, even taking the girlfriend with him on visits at the nursing home. Can you imagine the effect this had on early stage AD patients such as Sue who watched the video?

Each person with AD exhibits different symptoms, but the overall result is the same. In Sue and PJ's case, their common symptoms are:

1. Frustration when people don't believe the diagnosis
2. Vision problems
3. Embarrassed at social gaffs
4. Problems with numbers
5. Lapses in memory; deep concern about time

In addition, Sue becomes disoriented in a new setting, is ignored in conversation, and has spatial issues, while PJ is concerned about sleep problems, loneliness, and depression.

THOSE WITHOUT FAMILY SUPPORT

Sue and PJ have the support of their family and friends, but what happens to people who lack that support? In a bad economy, with a shortage of social workers, some people fall through the cracks. Before my husband showed signs of Alzheimer's and before Sue told me she had Alzheimer's, my husband was manager of a large apartment complex. I found myself involved on two occasions with older tenants who had no family nearby and showed definite signs of dementia. I was able to find assistance for them both, but, as in most cases where government social programs come into play, it took several months to get help.

I presently live in an assisted living facility, having moved here with my husband a few years ago and now living alone. It seems there is always a tenant who lives alone and shows signs of dementia but has no help. If that is the case in an apartment complex, how many others are living alone in a private home and desperately need help? The decision to move someone into a nursing home is especially difficult for family members, who feel that they are giving up. In the support group I attended before David died, there were several caregivers who were being torn apart by guilt because they had put their loved one into a nursing home.

Those with Alzheimer's exhibit different symptoms, but one of the most difficult is the patient who simply refuses to accept this new lifestyle and never lets family forget how much they hate being in a nursing home. One such case was a husband in a support group who was exhibiting signs of dementia himself and just couldn't understand why he couldn't take care of his wife at home; another was a daughter whose mother just didn't understand how her daughter could do this to her and never stopped letting her know it. The guilt can be overwhelming. David had already had a taste of nursing homes when we returned from Mexico, and because at that time it was temporary, he didn't like it but he made the best of it. The night before he died, however, I had decided it was time. I had to call 911 to help put him in bed. I simply couldn't manage him myself. He was a big man. The guilt I felt wasn't because I was going to send him to a nursing home; it was that I wasn't fulfilling my caregiver role. The fact that he died the next morning compounded the guilt, but I know now that it would have been the best thing for both of us if he had gone to a nursing home earlier.

BIBLIOGRAPHY

Dienstag, Alan. 2010. "Lessons from the Lifelines Writing Group for People in the Early Stages of Alzheimer's Disease: Forgetting What We Don't Remember." *Public Radio.* http://being .publicradio.org/programs/2010/alzheimers/essay_dienstag-. lessonsfromthelifelines.shtml.

Peterson, Barry. 2010. *Jan's Story.* California: Behler. Lake Forest, CA: Behler Publications.

9

Where Do We Go from Here?

SHARING THE NEWS

Sue and PJ were invited to speak at an Elder Law Clinic (ELC) seminar at Syracuse University in 2010. They were joined by PJ's daughter, Tiffany Riihinen, and Ellen Somers, MA, coordinator of Cognitive Health Services and a board member of the Alzheimer's Association, Central New York Chapter.

PJ offered humor in her remarks, introducing herself by saying, "Dementia is so much fun [pause—wry smile] but I don't recommend it." She went on to speak about her awareness of the disease, which often leads to depression, "but," she said, "I would rather have depression because it means I have enough marbles to play the game." Sue was more matter-of-fact. "This is what was given to me. It's not great, but at least we know."

The students asked Sue and PJ questions about their mental and physical capacity and drafting powers of attorney, health care proxies, and wills and trusts. Both understand the need for such documents, but they leave it to Sue's husband, Gary, and PJ's husband, Bob, to take care of those types of legal affairs. In the meantime, they both have a strong desire to remain connected and contribute to their community as long as they can.

For family and friends, it would be helpful if the person either diagnosed with Alzheimer's disease (AD) or thinking they might have it could articulate how they personally feel about the disease by answering the following questions:

1. Have you been diagnosed or is it still only a possibility? How long did it take to be diagnosed?
2. What were your earliest experiences and symptoms that you didn't understand?
3. How did your family react to the diagnosis?
4. Are you still working?
5. Do you know others with early stage?
6. Do you take Aricept and Namenda? Do they help?
7. Do you have relatives nearby or do they live elsewhere?
8. Have you accepted the diagnosis or the possible diagnosis?
9. Have you established a routine that works for you?

FINANCIAL ASSISTANCE

Caregivers and family members usually make decisions about finances, but it is recommended that the patient be included in the decision-making steps, at least being given the option to offer suggestions on how they feel, even though it might not change the overall process. Advance planning is necessary, and the patient should be included in the planning as much as possible. Most of the burden for care of AD patients is met by individuals and families, not Medicare or Medigap insurance.

Perhaps the most important decision to be made is whether to sign up for long-term care (LTC) insurance when a diagnosis is suspected but not given, finding out what is covered and when benefits could start being collected. Does it cover home care as well as nursing home care? This is the time when a blood test that predicts the possibility of AD in the future would allow someone to sign up for LTC insurance long before symptoms show up. AD causes a gradual decline in cognitive abilities from the time it is diagnosed to the time patients are in the final stages. Therefore, financial assistance is needed over a number of years. Social Security Disability Insurance (SSDI) is possible for those under 65, even though it is only a small percentage of previous earned income. In February 2010, "the Social Security Administration added early onset Alzheimer's to the list of conditions under its Compassionate Allowance Initiative, giving those with the disease expedited access to SSDI and Supplemental Security Income (SSI)." The National Clearinghouse for Long-Term Care Information is a government site that presents the different types of LTC as well as how to plan and pay for the care.

Because of AD's progressive nature, SSDI notes that different types of care require different costs that might need to be faced:

1. Ongoing medical treatment, including diagnosis and follow-up visits
2. Treatment for other medical conditions
3. Prescription drugs
4. Personal care supplies
5. Adult supportive day programs
6. In-home care services
7. Residential care services
8. Social services

CULTURAL ASPECTS OF AD

After a diagnosis of AD, family members and friends have trouble accepting the diagnosis because in early stages others can't really see any change to speak of. Only a caregiver who spends every day with the disease notices the differences. Some of the early changes for Sue and PJ were disorientation in a new setting, spatial issues, embarrassment at social gaffs, problems with numbers, deep concern about time, loneliness, and depression. David was in mid-stage AD and for him it was hallucinations, obsessing, up at night, loss of appetite, lack of balance, incontinence, drastic mood swings, disoriented about time, and not knowing if it was day or night.

As noted by the Alzheimer's Update site, the extent to which a person with AD can make simple or complex decisions depends on personality and progression of the disease. Caregivers are apt to take over decision-making and not give a person with AD an opportunity to contribute thoughts on ways to deal with the disease and future life style. When this happens, it is very possible that some caregivers might put their own interests first.

It has been almost five years since Sue was diagnosed and longer since PJ received her diagnosis. Perhaps the most important discovery has been how lonely these women were before they met each other. For those with early onset AD, communicating with others who also have the disease is very important. Unfortunately, very few support groups are set up for early onset AD patients. There are several reasons why it is difficult to organize a group of early stage patients—one reason is that it takes so long to come up with a diagnosis in those younger than 65. Another reason is that the belief that those with Alzheimer's cannot communicate is a common belief. Even when told a person has early onset AD, there is a lack of acceptance that the person has the disease.

Accepting the limitations brought about by AD is difficult but imperative. It is necessary to avoid stressful situations. As the disease progresses, it takes more and more time to complete a common task. When in the company of those whose thinking is not impaired, it becomes obvious those people don't understand what is happening. They become impatient and you become frustrated. AD is a disease that changes your daily routine. Glenn Campbell, award-winning country singer, was diagnosed with Alzheimer's, but he continued his career after diagnosis with a new album and singing engagements with his children as backup on stage. He is now retired from singing publicly and often forgets that he has Alzheimer's, but he and his family have established a routine that works for them.

Unfortunately, a possible symptom of Alzheimer's for those over 65 or in the later stages is violent behavior. This often manifests itself when the patient is faced with changes that take away the familiar, the routine they've been following for quite some time. The diagnosis of Alzheimer's in older people usually comes after they have been showing symptoms for years. By the time the diagnosis is made, the patient is out of the loop and simply knows that life has changed but doesn't know why. They have difficulty processing the diagnosis, knowing only that they are facing the unknown and they fight the efforts of others to make them conform to a new routine.

One of the difficulties faced with Dave was the many changes of residence over the last year of his life. He began to have hallucinations and would sometimes become angry when too many changes occurred in a short time. From the time we decided we had to return to Massachusetts until we ultimately moved into an extended-care apartment, Dave was hospitalized in San Diego in August for a week, spent the night after discharge from the hospital in a motel, traveled to San Diego airport, changed planes twice, was back in the hospital for another week in Pittsfield, then to a nursing home, and finally to an apartment, where we stayed from October 2008 to March 2009, with one more hospital stay. Is it any wonder he suffered from hallucinations and became angry and discouraged much of the time in his last few weeks?

I have to say that if Dave had lived longer than he did and had gone to a nursing home, it would have been the best I could do for him and for me. First of all, I would have applied for Medicaid, since we had little financial security and I could be assured that Dave was taking his medication properly. This was not the case at home because he was up at night while I was asleep. At the nursing home, he would have had access to a shower and to food and drinks that he liked. We had a tub shower that he had trouble getting in and out of and so he refused to bathe at home. At the nursing home, he would have a scheduled day with exercise, going to the game room, walking in the halls, staying up at night to engage with the night staff, and once in a while having a beer.

I agree that not all nursing homes are as attuned to the needs of patients as they should be, and it is unfortunate that the public perception is so negative, because Alzheimer's is a disease that just continues to progress, and the time will come when a caregiver cannot do it alone anymore, no matter how much they want to.

If anyone thinks health care in the United States is not a huge concern, just look at the 5.4 million people with AD and related incurable dementias, who will require constant care from diagnosis to death. The numbers of early onset patients who have had to give up their jobs and their plans for retirement are at present trying to deal with this costly disease that will eventually require constant care without the funds to allow any respite for caregivers. If we look at the impact of increasing cases of AD in American society as compared with other major illnesses, regardless of what percentage of the population is confronted with Alzheimer's, it will eventually comprise the largest concern, and only with a cure can it be contained.

LATEST IN ALZHEIMER'S RESEARCH STUDIES

The two major medications used in the treatment of AD are Aricept and Namenda. These medications have been around for a number of years, and although there might be side effects, the early benefits make them acceptable. According to a recent editorial by Peter Berger in *Alzheimer's Weekly*, "researchers have found that these two medications lead all other therapies by a wide margin in the treatment of newly diagnosed AD patients."

The Alzheimer's Drug Discovery Foundation (ADDF) and the Lewy Body Dementia Association (LBDA) have joined to generate the discovery of innovative biomarkers that aid in early diagnosis, detection and disease monitoring of Lewy Body dementia (LBD), and Parkinson's dementia. Many individuals who have LBD are misdiagnosed, most commonly with Alzheimer's or Parkinson's diseases. Developing effective biomarkers such as those in a blood test that cannot only predict AD, but what type, is key to correctly diagnosing the disease and eventually curing LBD and other dementias.

ULTIMATE GOALS IN RESEARCHING AD

A recent draft by the U.S. Department of Health and Human Resources for a national plan to address AD was presented online for public discussion. While the ultimate goal is to develop effective prevention and treatment modalities, research and clinical inquiry now can increase our ability to delay the onset of AD, minimize the symptoms, and delay progression.

As of January 2012, this national plan, the National Alzheimer's Project Act, was signed and provides the opportunity to create tools for early detection and effective therapies for AD. The Act sets forth a timeline for effective prevention and treatment for Alzheimer's by 2025, which, according to Rachel Doody of Baylor University, would prioritize and accelerate scientific research; however, it doesn't offer the way in which that research could be utilized. Another aspect of the plan recognizes the need for properly educated direct care workers, physicians, and other health professionals, but doesn't go on to say how these workers would be motivated to obtain this type of education. Moody suggests a network of memory disorders centers, where actual treatment could take place. The plan is also generally responsive to the needs of families in terms of support, but the services offering this support have decreased budgets rather than increased financing, and there are many day-in, day-out problems that need to be addressed, such as transportation, since it is standard practice for doctors to tell their Alzheimer's patients not to drive. A major goal is to enhance public awareness by providing tools to everyone who interacts with patients to help them identify signs of cognitive impairment and acceleration of the disease.

The overall plan is a worthy effort toward comprehensive reform, and the perspectives of Alzheimer's patients, their families, and the providers who also care for them create a chief unifying theme across the network of goals. In May 2012, the National Institute on Aging (NIA) initiated a research summit, open to the public. National and international experts in AD and dementia offer information about clinical trials on pharmacologic and non-pharmacologic ways to prevent, manage, and treat AD.

Enrollment in these trials is very much encouraged. In the meantime, some of the priorities in educating the public about research findings are noted as follows:

1. Promising findings should be highlighted with additional steps taken to expand knowledge to the general public, medical practitioners, industry, and public health systems.
2. High-quality care should be available from point of diagnosis through end-of-life and in settings such as people's homes, doctors' offices, hospitals, and nursing homes, with the specialist training needed.
3. Diagnosis of AD or related dementias needs to be made before symptoms become severe. Research has identified some assessment tools that will help health care providers make a diagnosis early in the disease.
4. For patients and families dealing with AD, especially for those with early-stage AD, counseling, support, or information about the next steps to be taken should be instituted.
5. Caregivers need information and training that will help them prepare for the challenges they will face in caring for an Alzheimer's patient. Families need help to plan for potential LTC.
6. Finally, people with AD deserve to be treated with dignity. Education of the general public about AD will help them understand how to best interact with those who have the disease.

EARLY DIAGNOSIS

A diagnosis of AD is devastating, but if it can be made in its earliest stages, everyone concerned, both patient and family, can set up a life plan to meet the challenges as the disease progresses. The hope is to find a cure for this disease as time goes on.

Research in 2012 has increased substantially as the numbers of people with some type of dementia continues to grow. The "baby boomers" are now in their 50s and increased population will no doubt greatly expand the numbers of Alzheimer's patients, especially those in the early stages. Although a cure is still not available, the focus now is on finding ways to determine whether a person might be at risk for AD before cognitive symptoms have manifested themselves.

Research suggests that a combination of the metabolic rate in the brain as measured by Positron Emission Tomography (PET) scans and genetic risk factors may be one way to detect AD before symptoms are evident. Another study used Magnetic Resonance Imaging (MRI) to follow participants over a three-year period, and researchers found they could identify those at risk for the disease with a high degree of accuracy.

For those who are found to be at risk for AD before any symptoms are present, this knowledge may be difficult to accept. Some steps could be taken to prepare for a future illness that may or may not happen, but the question that arises is whether someone wants to know ahead of time that the risk is there. Anyone who has a family member with AD already wonders if they are more susceptible. When they see no signs in themselves, it's much easier to avoid testing and dismiss the possibility. Therefore, that will be a future concern as research continues.

At present, two screening tools are recommended for physicians to use as a way to determine cognitive difficulties:

1. Mini mental status exam—Tests a person's orientation, attention, calculations, recall, language, and motor skills.
2. Memory Impairment Screen—A four-item recall test that assesses memory impairment.

The burden of caring for Alzheimer's patients will continue to fall largely on primary care physicians because there is a lack of specialists in this field. Based on findings of neurologist Dr. John Morris, writer Alice Park of *Time* presents the downside of new diagnostic criteria that would reclassify mild AD as mild cognitive impairment (MCI). Not all patients diagnosed with MCI go on to have Alzheimer's, although almost all cases of Alzheimer's start with MCI. The treatments for those with Alzheimer's are more effective in the early stages of the disease, but medications available so far, such as Aricept and Namenda, are only moderately beneficial over time. Namenda is usually prescribed in more advanced cases of Alzheimer's and not early stage AD. In my husband's case,

Namenda was added to his medications, but unfortunately all it did was make him almost catatonic, and we had to stop giving it to him.

More focus is being given by experts on early stage AD, and treatment that is not really helpful for advanced cases of AD is being shown to specifically benefit early stages of the disease. Doctors need to spend more time with patients who show signs of cognitive impairment, rather than making a decision based on one visit with a battery of tests. Whether or not the doctor chooses to diagnose MCI when the impairment has little effect on every-day life—the patient might have difficulty paying bills, doing taxes, or cooking when these problems didn't previously exist—the result is confusing to the patient who knows something is wrong but not why. Doctors hesitate to mention the possibility of dementia because of its negative image, but family members need to be included in an ongoing study to determine which diagnosis is the most likely. A diagnosis of MCI, which doesn't seem as bad as dementia, can cause concern for those who actually have early stage AD and for the doctor who hesitates to name Alzheimer's as the culprit. This is why monitoring over a period of time is needed; treatment can be started regardless of when an actual diagnosis can be made. Fortunately, the present success of a blood test that can predict dementia before symptoms appear offers a way to indicate whether a patient is susceptible to AD as time goes on. There is no way to know just when this blood test can be used as a tool, but the results look good. The bottom line, of course, is to find a cure, and with the increased attention on the disease, more time and money can be spent on doing just that. The number of people diagnosed with dementia is presently 5.4 million, but when those considered to have MCI are added, the number increases by 3 million for a total of 8.4 million, which is 5% of the total population of the United States.

ALZHEIMER'S IN A GLOBAL SOCIETY

Although this book focuses on Alzheimer's in the United States, the disease definitely has a global impact and the non-profit organization, Alzheimer's Disease International (ADI), in its 2010 report called for action on the part of governments and policy makers across the world to address this disease. The report encourages increased emphasis on lack of recognition of dementia in low-income countries, as well as the societal cost worldwide. Alzheimer's International states that, as of 2010, 35.6 million people were living with dementia and the prediction is that this number will increase to 65.7 million by 2030 and 115.4 million by 2050, mostly occurring in low- and middle-income countries.

According to the 2010 report, "there is an urgent need to develop cost-effective packages of medical and social care that meet the needs of people with dementia and their caregivers across the course of the illness and evidence-based prevention strategies." The cost of dementia globally is the highest in the North America High Income Groups and Western Europe, with 21 regional areas represented.

Worldwide, the costs of dementia are set to soar and the United States leads in this area. "Recently published data from the UK suggests that a 15-fold increase [in funding for Alzheimer's] is required to reach parity with research into heart disease and a 30-fold increase to achieve parity with cancer." Only by investing now in research and cost-effective approaches to care can future societal costs be anticipated and managed on a global basis.

Key activities are (1) global awareness; (2) training and education in running a non-profit organization; (3) hosting an international conference; (4) offering reliable and accurate information through web sites and publications; and 5) supporting the 10/66 Dementia Research Groups and their work on impact of dementia in developing countries. That 10/66 refers to the two-thirds (66%) of people with dementia living in low- and middle-income countries, and the 10% or less of population-based research that has been carried out in those regions.

Health care at present is organized around an acute episodic model of care that no longer meets the need of patients with chronic conditions. Worldwide ADI calls on governments to institute policies and plans for LTC that support family and caregivers and protect vulnerable people living with dementia.

The societal cost of dementia is already enormous and economic impact on families is insufficiently appreciated. A survey covering adults in the United States, Germany, France, Spain, and Poland found that more people would seek medical advice if they developed symptoms of AD and would likely get a test (if such a test existed, which to date does not). Only about 40% of survey respondents realized that AD is a fatal condition. The survey also indicated that many think there is an effective treatment to slow the symptoms and the progression (but so far, there is not). Only in the United States did a majority (61%) register a clear concern about the disease's ability to end a life.

Lower income countries face a heavy burden on families and caregivers who have no knowledge of what is happening to loved ones suffering from dementia. The most key decision makers must take notice and make dementia a national and global health priority. It would bide well for the United States to at least consider global health plans, since our present system often doesn't cover the needs of American citizens who live in poverty and can't afford medical care, especially those with dementia or other forms of incurable illness. The total estimated worldwide costs of dementia were $604 billion in 2010, increasing through 2011 and into 2012.

UNITED STATES RANKS LAST IN HEALTH CARE WORLDWIDE

In a 2010 health care study, the United States was compared to six other countries—Britain, Canada, Germany, the Netherlands, Australia, and New Zealand—and was ranked in last place. In most developed countries, health care is paid for largely by the government or an organization associated with it, using taxes collected from citizens. Britain, with a "single-payer" health plan, ranks first in quality, while in the United States a portion of the health care system is market-based with government-provided Medicare and Medicaid (covering those over 65 and those living in poverty). Care in the mainstream is generally delivered by private organizations and individuals, and all parts of the system are subject to some level of competition.

Because of the competitive nature of health care coverage in the United States, those who have been diagnosed with Alzheimer's might not have a policy that covers LTC, and no doubt will be denied long-term insurance coverage by private companies. Making a decision to sign up for LTC insurance at an early age, when there is no way to know if dementia of some kind is in the future, is difficult. The policy should have riders to protect against inflation and pay an additional amount to have the home renovated to accommodate someone with Alzheimer's, if necessary. Sue and Gary have had to make renovations to their home, but they don't have long-term coverage.

Health care reform includes the Community Living Assistance Services Act (CLASS Act) and all Americans will have access to this coverage. They will be enrolled automatically into an LTC insurance program and can opt out of the coverage if they want. No medical screening is necessary and premium payments will last five years and can be deducted from payroll. A cash payment will pay for home care and people can enjoy up to 50% discount on prescription drugs. The above information would seem to be beneficial and for some it is, but this program is only available to those who are still working and can afford to pay the premiums for five years before LTC is needed. Therefore, Sue and PJ aren't able to sign up for LTC since they cannot work. For those whose net worth is less than $300,000, LTC is not a good buy. No more than 5% of income should be spent on a LTC policy. For those who ultimately need LTC insurance but have few financial resources, the option at present is Medicaid.

In an interview with David Hyde Pierce (TV celebrity), who has been involved in fund raising for the Alzheimer's Association for 15 years, Pierce notes that while funding for most major diseases is in the billions, Alzheimer's is in the millions. The National Institutes of Health spends about $450 million a year on dementia research. Earlier this year, the Obama administration announced it would add an extra $50 million to that tab this year, and seek $80 million more to spend on Alzheimer's research in 2013.

HOPE SPRINGS ETERNAL

According to Richard Alleyne, science correspondent for *The Telegraph* in Great Britain, researchers have been able to detect "markers" in the blood that identify AD three to five years before any memory loss occurs. Along with the growing focus on the disease, with national and international studies offering a platform for the public in 2012, these findings increase the possibility of early diagnosis. Treatment could be started before irreversible brain damage has occurred. In the meantime, those who have already been diagnosed can make every effort to establish a lifestyle that will slow the progression of the disease and allow for the possibility that there will be a cure.

For Sue and PJ, the disease is something they are living with every day, but by writing this book with me over the past year and a half, they have not only exercised their brains, but have fulfilled their desire to educate people about what it is like to have AD by those who have it.

BIBLIOGRAPHY

Alzheimer's Disease Education and Referral Center. 2010. "Participating in Alzheimer's Disease Clinical Trials and Studies Fact Sheet." NIH Publication No. 09-7484. http://www.nia.nih.gov/Alzheimers/Publications/trials-studies.html.

Alz.org. 2011. "Draft Framework for the Plan to Address Alzheimer's Disease." http://napa.alz.org/share-your-feedback.

Associated Press. 2012. "US Alzheimer's Strategy: Better Treatment by 2025, Earlier Diagnosis and Caregiver Help Sooner." http://www.washingtonpost.com/national/health-science/us-alzheimers-strategy-better-treatment-by-2025-earlier-diagnosis-and-caregiver-help-sooner/2012/02/22/gIQAyhBlTR_story.html.

Berger, Peter, ed. "Good Decisions by People with Dementia." *Alzheimer's Weekly.com* Updated October 16, 2011.

Berger, Peter, ed. "Doctors Prefer Aricept and Amenda for Alzheimer's." *Alzheimer's Weekly.com*, June 11, 2012. http://alzheimersweekly.com/content/doctors-prefer-aricept-namenda-alzheimers.

Dienstag, Alan. 2010. "Lessons from the Lifelines Writing Group for People in the Early Stages of Alzheimer's Disease: Forgetting What We Don't Remember." *Public Radio*. http://being.publicradio.org/programs/2010/alzheimers/essay_dienstag-lessonsfromthelifelines.shtml.

Doody, Rachelle S. 2012. "The National Alzheimer's Plan: An Opportunity For Action." *Kaiser Health News*. http://www.kaiserhealthnews.org/stories/2012/january/30/different-takes-dr-doody.aspx.

Park, Alice. 2012. "New Criteria May Change Alzheimer's Diagnosis." *Time*. http://healthland.time.com/2012/02/08/why-a-new-definition-of-cognitive-impairment-may-confuse-patients/.

Robakis, Daphne, and Susan Donaldson, James. 2012. "Alzheimer's Disease: 3 Million More Americans Should Get Diagnosis, Study Concludes." *Alzheimer's News*. http://abcnews.go.com/Health/AlzheimersNews/alzheimers-disease-million-americans-diagnosis-study-concludes/story?id=15522248.

Social Security Update. 2009. "Outreach Hearing on Alzheimer's and Related Dementias: Compassionate Allowances." http://www.socialsecurity.gov/newsletter/archives/2009/july2009.html.

Strauch, Jesse, Interviewer. 2011. "David Hyde Pierce: Raising Awareness About Alzheimer's." *NBC News*, Updated October 19, 2011. http://www.msnbc.msn.com/id/44966598/ns/us_news-giving/t/david-hyde-pierce-raising-awareness-about-alzheimers/.

"World Alzheimer Report 2010: the Global Economic Impact of Dementia - Executive Summary." Alzheimer's Disease International (ADI). UK: London. http://www.alz.co.uk/research/world-report.

Appendix

I took care of a lady with Alzheimer's years ago, becoming her conservator and helping her find a nursing home. Below is the article I wrote for The Berkshire Eagle *published on March 11, 1990. After 22 years, the same problems exist, with an increased population suffering from some form of dementia, mostly Alzheimer's.*

GROWING OLD: INDEPENDENCE FADES

By Marjorie N. Allen
Reprinted with permission
© *The Berkshire Eagle*, Pittsfield, MA

Charlie Peck made sure his wife, Marie, had enough assets to live on the interest if anything happened to him. But Charlie couldn't anticipate before he died 16 years ago that Marie might become confused and have trouble remembering just how much money she had or where it might be. And he couldn't know that there would be no family left to take care of her affairs; nor that she either needed to be exceptionally wealthy or completely destitute before any agency, public or private, would give her a second thought.

Marie is 85 years old now, and because she has an income that generates enough interest to put her above the minimum threshold for Medicaid, the state considers her "private pay," and its hands, according to a spokeswoman, are "tied."

The state can't become involved in her care. Only when her savings are used up and she is entirely dependent on Social Security will she be eligible for Medicaid. That won't take long in a state-run nursing home, which charges $120 a day. On the other hand, she would need at least half a million dollars in income-producing assets before she could afford private-pay nursing home care for an unlimited period of time.

Marie may be 85, but her physical health is exceptionally good. She had measles and chicken pox during her childhood and has never needed medical care throughout her adult life—until now. Because she might be in the beginning stages of Alzheimer's disease—the symptoms began about four years ago—she needs custodial care. That's another way of saying nursing home care.

CHANGES IN ROUTINE

No more walks to Newberry's on North Street. No more trips to the A&P and back when she needs a few groceries. And as much as she likes to walk, as she clings to her independence, she hasn't been going out so often because she's apt to get lost and wander about for several hours, and she gets very tired. It's also pretty cold these days to be walking to Newberry's, with the wind whistling down North Street—she keeps forgetting that she has a warm coat and wears her thin spring coat that is becoming spotted and worn.

She leaves her gas stove on with no pilot light, and she forgets to pay her cable and telephone bills. "The cable man is here to disconnect your cable, Marie," I say. "If I write the check, will you sign it?" She signs it, and the cable man offers to send the bill to me, her neighbor, next time.

The term "nursing home" in the past has created an image of residents in a state of despair. That is less the case now, with new awareness of the problems of the elderly, but in many nursing homes, there is still a lineup, a group of people sometimes but not always in wheelchairs, seated all in a row next to the nursing station, people with blank faces and hopeless eyes. "I don't like this place," Marie says of such a nursing home, one of the many we visited. "You know my friend Alma? We went to high school together. Why can't I live where she lives, next to the museum?"

"You don't have enough money," I answer.

"Not enough money," she murmurs, her eyes tragic.

But all nursing homes aren't the same. Berkshire Hills North in Lee doesn't have a lineup. It's a beehive of activity, and you can feel its pulse the moment you walk in the door. People are playing games, chatting, reading. Many are in wheelchairs, but they're busy traveling through the halls. The nursing station is the hub of a wheel with corridors creating the spokes.

After Charlie died in 1974, Marie moved from Canandaigua, NY, to Lee, MA, where she had friends, and then to Pittsfield. She prefers Lee. And Berkshire Hills North is close enough to Main Street to suit her. But she suddenly realizes that in this facility she'll have to share a room after many years of being by herself. It's another adjustment in a long list of adjustments confronting this woman who is trying her best to deal with a world that in the last few years too often eludes her. Her only relative, a cousin, suffered a stroke a few years earlier and is under the complete care of his wife. "Charlie was an only child, and so was I," she says.

Recently, Marie and I gathered together the things she cared about the most—pictures of her mother, an easy chair, two straight back chairs, a small table and her clothing. She loves pink. Almost everything she has is pink. And after a going-away party at the apartment complex, she made the move to Lee. It wasn't an easy decision, but when the call came that there was an opening, there was no time to dwell on it. The decision had to be made.

Marie's confusion has caused her at times to express some paranoia, but on the whole she is secure in her new home. A tabby cat sleeps on her bed, and her belongings from home create a cozy corner. But she worries about the cost. "I don't need all this room," she says, convinced she's renting the whole facility. She wears a bracelet that sets off an alarm if she tries to leave the building. Only when someone accompanies her can she go outside.

I took her to Johansson's in downtown Lee, and she browsed through the variety store. She found a sweater she liked—pink. When we returned to the nursing home, she said, "This is within walking distance of the stores, isn't it?"

"Yes, it is," I answer. I don't have the heart to remind her that she can't go by herself.

CLINGING TO INDEPENDENCE

She still clings to her independence. Dr. Robert Wespiser, the nursing home physician, says it is important to keep the residents open to the world around them and to correct physical problems whenever possible.

"You have cataracts, Marie," he tells her during her initial exam. "If you had an operation, you could see better."

"I can see just fine!" she snaps back.

"No rush," he says. "We'll talk later."

She said the last time I visited her, "I'd like to get a small flat on Main Street. They won't let me leave this place."

It's a terrible struggle to maintain dignity in the face of such changes. "You're 85 now, Marie," I explain. "You can't do the things you used to do."

"I know," she answers. "I know."

Glossary

Acetylcholine—A neurotransmitter that appears to be involved in learning and memory. Acetylcholine is severely diminished in Alzheimer's disease.

Alzheimer's disease (AD)—A progressive, neurodegenerative disease characterized by loss of function and death of nerve cells in several areas of the brain leading to loss of cognitive function such as memory and language. The cause of nerve cell death is unknown. Alzheimer's disease is the most common cause of dementia.

Anxiety—A feeling of apprehension, fear, nervousness, or dread accompanied by restlessness or tension.

Aphasia—Difficulty understanding the speech of others and/or expressing oneself verbally.

Art therapy—A form of therapy that allows people with dementia to express their feelings creatively through art.

Behavioral symptoms—In Alzheimer's disease, the symptoms that relate to action or emotion, such as wandering, depression, anxiety, hostility, and sleep disturbances.

Brain—One of the two components of the central nervous system, the brain is the center of thought and emotion. It is responsible for the coordination and control of bodily activities, and the interpretation of information from the senses (sight, hearing, smell, etc.).

Caregiver—The primary person in charge of care of an Alzheimer's patient, usually a family member or a designated health care professional.

Cell—The fundamental unit of all organisms; the smallest structural unit that is capable of independent functioning.

Central nervous system (CNS)—One of the two major divisions of the nervous system. Composed of the brain and spinal cord, the CNS is the control center for the entire body.

Cerebral cortex—The outer portion of the brain, consisting of layers of nerve cells and the pathways that connect them. The cerebral cortex is the part of the brain in which thought processes take place. In Alzheimer's disease, nerve cells in the cerebral cortex die.

Cholinergic system—The system of nerve cells that uses acetylcholine as its neurotransmitter; nerve cells in the cholinergic system are damaged in the brains of Alzheimer's patients.

Clinical trial—Carefully controlled studies to test the value of various treatments, such as drugs or surgery for disease, in human beings.

Cognitive symptoms—Symptoms that relate to disorders in thought processes, such as learning, comprehension, memory, reasoning, and judging. These symptoms are prominent features of AD.

Creutzfeldt–Jakob disease—A rare disorder caused by prions that typically leads to rapid declines in memory and behavioral changes.

Deficits—Physical and/or cognitive skills or abilities that a person has lost, has difficulty with, or can no longer perform because of his or her dementia.

Dementia—Loss of intellectual functions (such as thinking, remembering, and reasoning) of sufficient severity to interfere within an individual's daily functioning.

Diagnosis—The process by which a doctor determines what disease a patient has by studying the patient's symptoms and medical history, and analyzing any tests performed (blood tests, urine tests, brain scans, etc.).

Differential diagnosis—The clinical evaluation of possible causes of dementia to rule out all other factors before settling on Alzheimer's disease as a diagnosis.

Disorientation—A cognitive disability in which the senses of time, direction, and recognition become difficult to distinguish.

Double-blind, placebo-controlled study—A research procedure in which neither researchers nor patients knows who is receiving the experimental substance or treatment and who is receiving a placebo.

Dysphasia—The inability to find the right word or understand the meaning of a word.

Early onset Alzheimer's disease—An unusual form of Alzheimer's disease in which individuals are diagnosed with the disease before age 65. Less than 10 percent of all Alzheimer's disease patients have early onset. Early onset Alzheimer's disease sometimes is associated with mutations in genes located on chromosomes 1, 14, and 21.

Early stage—The beginning stages of Alzheimer's disease when an individual experiences very mild to moderate cognitive impairments.

Hippocampus—A part of the brain that is important for learning and memory.

Informed consent—The agreement of a person (or his or her legally authorized representative) to serve as a research subject, in full knowledge of all anticipated risks and benefits of the experiment.

Late-onset Alzheimer's disease—The most common form of Alzheimer's disease, usually occurring after age 65. Late-onset Alzheimer's disease affects almost half of all people over the age of 85 and may or may not be hereditary.

Mild cognitive impairment (MCI)—A memory problem that is noticeable to others. People with MCI may have other problems in brain function as well, but they are able to get through the day and do what they need to do without major difficulty. Some (not all) people with MCI progress to develop Alzheimer's disease.

Multi-infarct dementia (MID)—Also known as vascular dementia, this form of dementia is caused by a number of strokes in the brain. These strokes can cause specific symptoms, depending on their severity and location, and can cause general symptoms of dementia. MID cannot be treated; once the nerve cells die, they cannot be replaced. However, the underlying condition leading to strokes (e.g., high blood pressure, diabetes) can be treated, which may help prevent further damage.

Nerve cell (neuron)—The basic working unit of the nervous system. The nerve cell is typically composed of a cell body containing the nucleus, several short branches (dendrites), and one long arm (the axon) with short branches along its length and at its end. Nerve cells send signals that control the actions of other cells in the body, such as muscle cells.

Neuritic plaque—Abnormal cluster of dead and dying nerve cells, other brain cells, and protein. Neuritic plaques are one of the characteristic structural abnormalities found in the brains of Alzheimer's patients. Upon autopsy, the presence of neuritic plaques and neurofibrillary tangles is used to positively diagnose AD.

Neurodegenerative disorder—A type of neurological disease marked by the loss of nerve cells. See Alzheimer's disease, Parkinson's disease.

Neurofibrillary tangle—Accumulation of twisted protein fragments inside nerve cells. Neurofibrillary tangles are one of the characteristic structural abnormalities found in the brains of Alzheimer's patients. Upon autopsy, the presence of neuritic plaques and neurofibrillary tangles is used to positively diagnose AD.

Neurological disorder—Disturbance in structure or function of the central nervous system resulting from developmental abnormality, disease, injury, or toxin.

Neurologist—A physician who diagnoses and treats disorders of the nervous system.

Neurotransmitter—Specialized chemical messenger (e.g., acetylcholine, dopamine, norepinephrine, serotonin) produced and secreted by nerve cells that sends a message from one nerve cell to another. Neurotransmitters play different roles throughout the body, many of which are not yet fully understood.

Nucleus—component of a cell containing all genetic material.

Prion—an infectious particle of protein that, unlike a virus, contains no nucleic acid, does not trigger an immune response, and is not destroyed by extreme heat or cold. These particles are considered responsible for such diseases as scrapie, bovine spongiform encephalopathy, kuru, and Creutzfeldt-Jakob disease.

Probable Alzheimer's disease—A level of diagnosis that is supported with relative certainty by the progressive deterioration of specific cognitive functions, motor skills and perception, impaired activities of daily living and altered patterns of behavior, as well as laboratory findings and brain scanning.

Repetitive behavior—Repeated questions, stories and outbursts, or specific activities done over and over again, common in people with dementia.

Side effect—An undesired effect of drug treatment that may range in severity from barely noticeable, to uncomfortable, to dangerous. Side effects are usually predictable.

Support group—A facilitated gathering of patients, caregivers, family, friends, or others affected by a disease or condition for the purpose of discussing issues related to the disease.

The above glossary was created from the two following sites:

- http://www.zarcrom.com/users/alzheimers/w7.html
- http://my.clevelandclinic.org/disorders/Alzheimers_Disease/hic_Alzheimers_Disease_Glossary_of_Terms.aspx

Resources

SUPPORT GROUPS

Sue and PJ are very interested in finding a way to involve patients as well as caregivers in showing their feelings about Alzheimer's. In support groups, both patients and caregivers participate, but there are all levels of Alzheimer's, with some who have lost their ability to communicate verbally. Priorities in a support group are to allow those who are verbal an opportunity to speak their thoughts. As noted earlier, the creative arts offer a base for communication with poetry, music, theater, and art projects.

Alan Dienstag's article on ways to improve the quality of life for Alzheimer's patients in a support group notes that it is one thing to have Alzheimer's at an older age, when health problems take precedence and Alzheimer-type symptoms are apt to be blamed on physical deterioration; these patients are either never told they have Alzheimer's or are unable to communicate whether they understand the implications of having the disease. Those with early onset, however, do know what the diagnosis means and have yet to lose their ability to communicate.

ORGANIZATIONS

Administration on Aging

The mission of Administration on Aging (AoA) is to develop a comprehensive, coordinated and cost-effective system of home and community-based services that helps elderly individuals maintain their health and independence in their homes and communities.
http://www.aoa.gov/AoARoot/About/index.aspx

Alzheimer's Disease Education and Referral Center

The Alzheimer's Disease Education and Referral (ADEAR) Center is a service of the federal government's National Institute on Aging (NIA), one of the National Institutes of Health (NIH). The Center provides accurate, up-to-date information about Alzheimer's disease (AD) and related disorders to patients and their families, caregivers, health care providers, and the public.
http://www.health.gov/nhic/nhicscripts/Entry.cfm?HRCode= HR2426

American Health Care Association

As the nation's largest association of long-term and post-acute care providers, American Health Care Association (AHCA) advocates for quality care and services for frail, elderly, and disabled Americans. Our members provide essential care to approximately one million individuals in 11,000 not-for-profit and proprietary member facilities.

American Society on Aging

The American Society on Aging (ASA) is an association of diverse individuals bound by a common goal: to support the commitment and enhance the knowledge and skills of those who seek to improve the quality of life of older adults and their families. The membership of ASA is multidisciplinary and inclusive of professionals who are

concerned with the physical, emotional, social, economic, and spiritual aspects of aging.
http://www.asaging.org/about-asa

Elder Care Online

This site offers a workbook to collect vital information off-line and use it at doctor's appointments.
http://www.ec-online.net/alzchannel.htm

Information Source for Adult Day Centers

Adult day service centers provide a coordinated program of professional and compassionate services for adults in a community-based group setting. They also afford caregivers respite from the demanding responsibilities of caregiving.

Medicare Rights Center

A not-for-profit organization that is the source for Medicare consumers and Medicare professionals.
http://www.medicarerights.org/about-mrc/

National Council on Aging

The National Council on Aging (NCOA) is a nonprofit service and advocacy organization headquartered in Washington, DC, a national voice for older Americans and the community organizations that serve them. We bring together nonprofit organizations, businesses, and government to develop creative solutions that improve the lives of all older adults.
http://www.ncoa.org/about-ncoa/

National Institutes of Health

The NIH, a part of the U.S. Department of Health and Human Services, is the nation's medical research agency—making important discoveries that improve health and save lives.
http://www.nih.gov/about/

SeniorResource.com

The "*E*-cyclopedia" of housing options and information for retirement, finance, insurance, and care.
http://www.seniorresource.com/

TRIALS AND STUDIES

Clinical studies observe people and help identify new possibilities for clinical trials. The NIA, part of the NIH, sponsors several major ongoing studies, including those on Alzheimer's disease.

Clinical trials for Alzheimer's patients are offered on a regular basis through the Internet. The effort is now going beyond a drug that slows symptoms to one that might act on some of the underlying causes of Alzheimer's. For those signing up for a trial, participants are divided into two groups, one taking the medication, the other taking a placebo. As long as the Alzheimer's patient can continue taking current medications, the placebo will not affect the patient's health, but those taking the research drug might either show progress or might have a negative reaction to the drug.

The Alzheimer's Association TrialMatch

By completing a questionnaire online or by phone, the Alzheimer's Association Contact Center will evaluate information and will contact the applicant as to whether he or she is eligible for a trial study.

Early-stage Alzheimer's is not related to age; early onset is. Even so, there is much to be learned from these people, who are willing to discuss their illness before they lose their ability to communicate.

Further Reading

ABC News Medical Unit. Accessed May 13, 2009. http://abcnews
.go.com/Health/AlzheimersNews/story?id=7571166&
page=1

Adams, Stephen. "Blood Test to Detect Early Stages of Alzheimer's."
The Telegraph. Accessed January 25, 2012. http://www
.telegraph.co.uk/health/healthnews/9039427/Blood-test-to-
detect-early-stages-of-Alzheimers.html

Alzheimer's Society of Canada. *Ethical Guidelines Alzheimer Care.*
Reviewed October 2005. http://www.alzheimer.ca/english/
care/ethics-decision.htm

Alzheimer'sTreatment.org. "Alzheimer's Care: Is it Time for an
Alzheimer's Nursing Home." ND. http://www.alzheimer-
streatment.org/care/nurshing.html

American Health Assistance Foundation. "Alzheimer's Treatments." Updated September 23, 2011. http://www.ahaf.org/
Alzheimers/treatment/common/

Axelson, Paul. "Oxidative Stress in Alzheimer's Disease." *American
Health Assistance Foundation.* July 1, 2011–June 30, 2013. http://
www.ahaf.org/research/grants/migrated/oxidative-lipid-
degradation.html

Burkholder, Amy. "Alzheimer's and the 'Silver Tsunami:' Is America
Ready?" *Health Blog.* CBS News. Accessed December 14, 2010.
http://www.cbsnews.com/8301-504763_162-20025655-
10391704.html

CBS Evening News. "Early Onset Alzheimer's On the Rise." *CBS News*. Accessed March 8, 2008. http://www.cbsnews.com/stories/2008/03/08/eveningnews/main3919747.shtml

Davis, Matt. "The Psychological Toll of Early Onset Alzheimer's Disease." *ABC News Medical Unit*. Accessed May 13, 2009. http://abcnews.go.com/Health/AlzheimersNews/story?id=7571166&page=1

DeBaggio, Thomas. 2002. *Losing My Mind: An Intimate Look at Life with Alzheimer's*. New York: Simon & Schuster.

Draper, Brian. 2004. *Dealing with Dementia: A Guide to Alzheimer's Disease and Other Dementias*, 5. Crows Nest, NSW: Allen & Unwin.

Fisher Center for Alzheimer's Research Foundation. 2010. "Alzheimer's Research on Diagnosis." http://www.alzinfo.org/research/alzheimers-research-on-diagnosis/

Fox, Maggie. "U.S. Scores Dead Last Again in Health Care Study." *Reuters*. Accessed June 23, 2010. http://www.reuters.com/article/2010/06/23/us-usa-healthcare-last-idUST-RE65M0SU20100623

Genova, Lisa. 2009. *Still Alice*. Pocket Books. New York: Simon & Schuster.

Glass, Jon. WebMD: Types of Dementia, 1–2. Accessed March 2, 2010. http://www.webmd.com/brain/types-dementia?page=1

Grohol, John M. "Survey Finds High Alzheimer's Awareness." *Psych Central*. Reviewed September 6, 2011. http://psychcentral.com/lib/2011/survey-finds-high-alzheimers-awareness/

History of Alzheimer's. *Alzheimer's Disease Research*. Accessed September 23, 2011. http://www.ahaf.org/alzheimers/about/understanding/history.html

Holt, G. Richard. 2011. "Timely Diagnosis and Disclosure of Alzheimer Disease Gives Patients Opportunities to Make Choices (September 2011)." *Southern Medical Journal* 104 (12).

Iliades, Chris. "Easing Alzheimer's Symptoms with Art Therapy." *Everyday Health.com*. Accessed January 14, 2009. http://www.everydayhealth.com/alzheimers/alzheimers-art-therapy.aspx

Kengor, Paul. "Reagan and Alzheimer's--What the Public Doesn't Know About the 40th President." *FoxNews.com*. Accessed January 18, 2011. http://www.foxnews.com/opinion/2011/01/18/reagan-alzheimers-public-doesnt-know-th-president/

King, James. 2010. *Bill Warrington's Last Chance*. New York: Viking.

Mobley, Tracy. 2007. *Young Hope: The Broken Road*. Parker, CO: Outskirts Press.

Moyer, Christine. "Reaching through the Fog: A Rising Tide of Alzheimer's Disease." *Amednews.* Accessed December 20, 2010. http://www.ama-assn.org/amednews/2010/12/20/prsa1220.htm

National Institute of Neurological Disorders and Stroke. "Creutzfeldt-Jakob Disease Fact Sheet." *National Institute of Health.* Updated December 28, 2011.

Peterson, Betsy. 2004. *Voices of Alzheimer's: Courage, Humor, Hope and Love in the Face of Dementia.* Cambridge, MA: Da Capo Press.

PubMed Health. 2011. National Center for Biotechnology Information. Bethesda, MD: U.S. National Library of Medicine. http://www.ncbi.nlm.nih.gov/pubmed/

Reaves, Jessica. "Trying Improv as Therapy for Those with Memory Loss." *Chicago News Cooperative.* Accessed August 7, 2010. http://www.chicagonewscoop.org/trying-improv-as-therapy-for-those-with-memory-loss/

Repko, Melissa. "After Early Alzheimer's Diagnosis, Flower Mount Couple Face Their Fears, Embrace Activism." *The Dallas Morning News.* Accessed November 28, 2010. http://www.dallasnews.com/health/medicine/20101128-after-early-alzheimer_s-diagnosis-flower-mound-.couple-face-their-fears-embrace-activism.ece

Sahelian, Ray. Natural Remedies for Alzheimer's Disease. http://www.raysahelian.com/alzheimer.html

Santich, Kate. "Poetry Project Helps Alzheimer's Patients Reconnect with Past, Present." *Orlando Sentinel.* Accessed July 5, 2010. http://articles.orlandosentinel.com/2010-07-05/news/os-alzheimers-poetry-project-20100705_1_poetry-readings-alzheimer-s-patients-participation

Shapiro, Joseph. *Alzheimer's Patients Struggle without Insurance.* NPR. Accessed July 6, 2009. http://www.npr.org/templates/story.php?storyId=106299147

Taylor, Glenda. "The Benefits of AARP." Accessed August 6, 2012. http://www.ehow.com/about_4617153_benefits-aarp.html

Taylor, Richard. 2007. *Alzheimer's from the Inside Out.* Baltimore: Health Professions Press.

Watson, Rita. "Alzheimer's and Dementia Mean Caregiver Stress for 15 Million." *Health News Examiner.* Accessed March 15, 2011. http://www.examiner.com/health-news-in-national/alzheimer-s-and-dementia-mean-caregiver-stress-for-15-million

Whitehouse, Peter, and Daniel George. 2008. *The Myth of Alzheimer's: What You Aren't Being Told About Today's Most Dreaded Diagnosis.* New York: St. Martin's Press.

Young, Ellen P. 1999. *Between Two Worlds: Special Moments of Alzheimer's and Dementia.* Amherst: Prometheus Books.

About the Authors

Marjorie N. Allen has published five children's books, including *Changes* (Simon & Schuster), *The Remarkable Ride of Israel Bissell As Related by Molly the Crow: Being the True Account of an Extraordinary Post Rider Who Persevered* (by Lippincott), and *One, Two, Three-Ah-Choo!* (Putnam). She has also published for adults, *What Are Little Girls Made of: A Guide to Female Role Models in Children's Books* and *One Hundred Years of Children's Books in America: Decade by Decade* (both published by Facts on File). Marjorie worked as a unit coordinator at Berkshire Medical Center in Pittsfield, MA, retiring after 10 years. She went to Smith College and still lives in Massachusetts. She was first introduced to Alzheimer's in 1990 after graduation from college, when her 85-year-old neighbor was showing signs of dementia and had no family to care for her. Marjorie helped her move to a nursing home where she spent the next ten years. Marjorie again was faced with Alzheimer's when her husband was diagnosed in 2008.

Susan Dublin has an RN/BS in Nursing and currently lives with her husband, Gary, in DeWitt, NY. Susan is in her early fifties and has been diagnosed with Alzheimer's disease. She has spoken widely on the topic in the area. She started her medical career after receiving a bachelor's degree in nursing from Hartwick College in Oneonta, NY. Her first job was at Crouse Irving Hospital in Syracuse, NY. She worked on a medical floor where she was a staff nurse, also in a rotation as charge nurse. She was office manager at

Linden Pediatrics in Syracuse, NY, for 19 years, leaving after she was diagnosed with Alzheimer's.

Patricia J. Kimmerly has a BS in secondary education from Parsons College of the University of Iowa, and an MS in Traumatic Brain Injury Rehab and Adult Education from Syracuse University. Her first professional job was teaching Junior High English and Speech in Kenosha, Wisconsin. She was co-founder of 4-county Planned Parenthood in Northern New York, worked with a CETA program in Ithaca, NY. She was Director of Education & Training at Cortland Memorial Hospital and Director of a residential facility for people with traumatic brain injury & cognitive disabilities in Washington, DC for National Rehab Hospital. She worked full time as faculty member for ILR school's program at Cornell University on Employment & Disability training, implementing the Americans with Disabilities Act all over the US.

Index